Health Wellness & Selfcare Journal

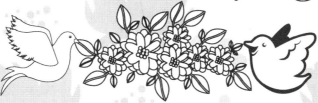

Personal Information

Name: _____

Address: _____

City/State/Zip: _____

Phone: _____

Cell: _____

Email: _____

Church: _____

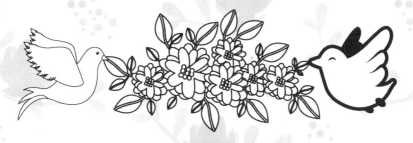

"For I know the plans I have for you," declares the LORD, "plans to prosper you and not to harm you, plans to give you hope and a future."

Jeremiah 29:11

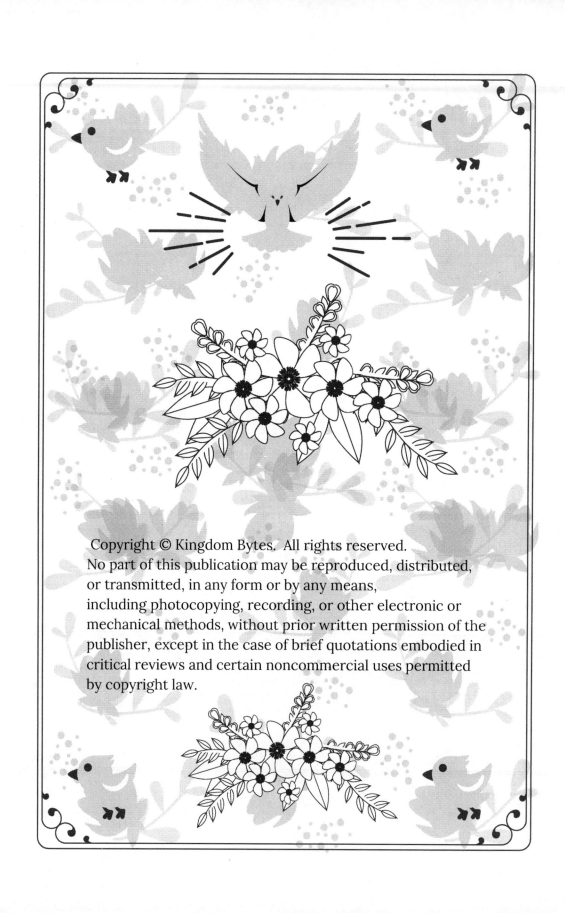

If anyone destroys God's temple, God will destroy him. For God's temple is holy,
and I am that temple. (1 Corinthians 3:17)

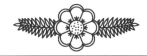

DAY 2	SU MO TU (WE) TH FR SA	How Do I Feel Today

DATE: _11-27-24_

BREAKFAST	LUNCH	DINNER

SNACKS:

A slimmer body is a gift from God, but
I still need to do the work! God does miracles
through the avenues he gives us!

TOTAL CALORIES	GLASSES OF WATER	HOURS OF SLEEP

WEIGHT	BLOOD PRESSURE	BLOOD SUGAR

EXERCISE/ PHYSICAL ACTIVITY	SELF-CARE ACTIVITY

I will present my body as a living sacrifice, holy and acceptable unto God, which is my spiritual worship. (Romans 12:1)

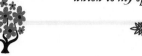 

DAY 3

SU MO TU WE TH FR SA

DATE: _____

How Do I Feel Today

BREAKFAST	LUNCH	DINNER

SNACKS:

TOTAL CALORIES	GLASSES OF WATER	HOURS OF SLEEP

WEIGHT	BLOOD PRESSURE	BLOOD SUGAR

EXERCISE/ PHYSICAL ACTIVITY	SELF-CARE ACTIVITY

I will not be conformed to this world, but will be transformed by the renewal of my mind; So that I will be able to test and approve what is God's good, pleasing and perfect will for my life.
(Romans 12:2)

 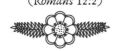

DAY 4

SU MO TU WE TH FR SA

DATE: _____

How Do I Feel Today

BREAKFAST	LUNCH	DINNER

SNACKS:

TOTAL CALORIES	GLASSES OF WATER	HOURS OF SLEEP

WEIGHT	BLOOD PRESSURE	BLOOD SUGAR

EXERCISE/ PHYSICAL ACTIVITY	SELF-CARE ACTIVITY

I will cast all my anxieties on Christ because he cares for me.
(1 Peter 5:7)

 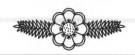

DAY 5	SU MO TU WE TH FR SA DATE: _____	How Do I Feel Today

BREAKFAST	LUNCH	DINNER

SNACKS:

TOTAL CALORIES	GLASSES OF WATER	HOURS OF SLEEP

WEIGHT	BLOOD PRESSURE	BLOOD SUGAR

EXERCISE/ PHYSICAL ACTIVITY	SELF-CARE ACTIVITY

You formed my inward parts, oh Lord; you knitted me together in my mother's womb.
I praise you, for I am fearfully and wonderfully made.   (Psalm 139:13-14)

 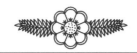

DAY 6	SU MO TU WE TH FR SA DATE: _____	How Do I Feel Today

BREAKFAST	LUNCH	DINNER

SNACKS:

TOTAL CALORIES	GLASSES OF WATER	HOURS OF SLEEP

WEIGHT	BLOOD PRESSURE	BLOOD SUGAR

EXERCISE/ PHYSICAL ACTIVITY	SELF-CARE ACTIVITY

I am fearfully and wonderfully made. Wonderful are your works; My soul knows that very well.
(Psalm 139:14)

DAY 7

SU MO TU WE TH FR SA

DATE: _____

How Do I Feel Today

BREAKFAST	LUNCH	DINNER

SNACKS:

TOTAL CALORIES	GLASSES OF WATER	HOURS OF SLEEP

WEIGHT	BLOOD PRESSURE	BLOOD SUGAR

EXERCISE/ PHYSICAL ACTIVITY	SELF-CARE ACTIVITY

I will clothe myself with the beauty that comes from within,
the unfading beauty of a gentle and quiet spirit which is so precious to God. (1 Peter 3:4)

 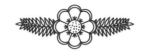

DAY 8

SU MO TU WE TH FR SA

DATE: _____

How Do I Feel Today

BREAKFAST	LUNCH	DINNER

SNACKS:

TOTAL CALORIES	GLASSES OF WATER	HOURS OF SLEEP

WEIGHT	BLOOD PRESSURE	BLOOD SUGAR

EXERCISE/ PHYSICAL ACTIVITY	SELF-CARE ACTIVITY

So then, there remains a Sabbath rest for the people of God, for whoever has entered God's rest has also rested from his works as God did from His. (Hebrews 4:9-10)

 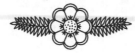

DAY 9

SU MO TU WE TH FR SA

DATE: _____

How Do I Feel Today

BREAKFAST	LUNCH	DINNER

SNACKS:

TOTAL CALORIES	GLASSES OF WATER	HOURS OF SLEEP

WEIGHT	BLOOD PRESSURE	BLOOD SUGAR

EXERCISE/ PHYSICAL ACTIVITY	SELF-CARE ACTIVITY

I will, make every effort to enter God's rest, so that I will not perish
by following an example of disobedience. (Hebrews 4:11)

 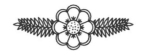

| DAY 10 | SU MO TU WE TH FR SA

DATE: _____ | How Do I Feel Today |

BREAKFAST	LUNCH	DINNER

SNACKS:

TOTAL CALORIES	GLASSES OF WATER	HOURS OF SLEEP

WEIGHT	BLOOD PRESSURE	BLOOD SUGAR

EXERCISE/ PHYSICAL ACTIVITY	SELF-CARE ACTIVITY

I will keep myself from being polluted by the world.
(James 1:27)

DAY 11

SU MO TU WE TH FR SA

DATE: _____

How Do I Feel Today

☐ ☐ ☐ ☐

BREAKFAST	LUNCH	DINNER

SNACKS:

TOTAL CALORIES	GLASSES OF WATER	HOURS OF SLEEP

WEIGHT	BLOOD PRESSURE	BLOOD SUGAR

EXERCISE/ PHYSICAL ACTIVITY	SELF-CARE ACTIVITY

I am God's masterpiece. He has created me anew in Christ Jesus, so that I can do the good things, which he planned for me long ago. (Ephesians 2:10)

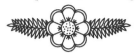

DAY 12

SU MO TU WE TH FR SA

DATE: _____

How Do I Feel Today

BREAKFAST	LUNCH	DINNER

SNACKS:

TOTAL CALORIES	GLASSES OF WATER	HOURS OF SLEEP

WEIGHT	BLOOD PRESSURE	BLOOD SUGAR

EXERCISE/ PHYSICAL ACTIVITY	SELF-CARE ACTIVITY

Physical training is good, but training for godliness is much better, promising benefits in this life and in the life to come. (1 Timothy 4:8)

 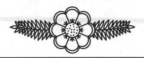

DAY 13	SU MO TU WE TH FR SA DATE: _____	How Do I Feel Today

BREAKFAST	LUNCH	DINNER

SNACKS:

TOTAL CALORIES	GLASSES OF WATER	HOURS OF SLEEP

WEIGHT	BLOOD PRESSURE	BLOOD SUGAR

EXERCISE/ PHYSICAL ACTIVITY	SELF-CARE ACTIVITY

I will seek the kingdom of God and his righteousness, and all things will be added to me.
(Matthew 6:33)

DAY 14	SU MO TU WE TH FR SA DATE: _____	How Do I Feel Today

BREAKFAST	LUNCH	DINNER

SNACKS:

TOTAL CALORIES	GLASSES OF WATER	HOURS OF SLEEP

WEIGHT	BLOOD PRESSURE	BLOOD SUGAR

EXERCISE/ PHYSICAL ACTIVITY	SELF-CARE ACTIVITY

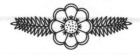

DAY 15

SU MO TU WE TH FR SA

DATE: _____

How Do I Feel Today

☐ ☐ ☐ ☐

BREAKFAST	LUNCH	DINNER

SNACKS:

TOTAL CALORIES	GLASSES OF WATER	HOURS OF SLEEP

WEIGHT	BLOOD PRESSURE	BLOOD SUGAR

EXERCISE/ PHYSICAL ACTIVITY	SELF-CARE ACTIVITY

The name of the Lord is a strong tower; the righteous run into it and are safe.
(Proverbs 18:10)

 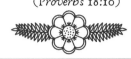

DAY 16	SU MO TU WE TH FR SA DATE: _____	How Do I Feel Today

BREAKFAST	LUNCH	DINNER

SNACKS:

TOTAL CALORIES	GLASSES OF WATER	HOURS OF SLEEP

WEIGHT	BLOOD PRESSURE	BLOOD SUGAR

EXERCISE/ PHYSICAL ACTIVITY	SELF-CARE ACTIVITY

Those who trust in the Lord, will lack no good thing. (Psalm 34:10)

 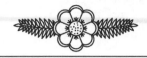

DAY 17	SU MO TU WE TH FR SA DATE: _____	How Do I Feel Today

BREAKFAST	LUNCH	DINNER

SNACKS:

TOTAL CALORIES	GLASSES OF WATER	HOURS OF SLEEP

WEIGHT	BLOOD PRESSURE	BLOOD SUGAR

EXERCISE/ PHYSICAL ACTIVITY	SELF-CARE ACTIVITY

The generous man will be prosperous, and he who waters, will himself be watered.
(Proverbs 11:25)

DAY 18	SU MO TU WE TH FR SA DATE: _____	How Do I Feel Today ☐ ☐ ☐ ☐

BREAKFAST	LUNCH	DINNER

SNACKS:

TOTAL CALORIES	GLASSES OF WATER	HOURS OF SLEEP

WEIGHT	BLOOD PRESSURE	BLOOD SUGAR

EXERCISE/ PHYSICAL ACTIVITY	SELF-CARE ACTIVITY

A man who is kind, benefits himself, but a cruel man hurts himself.
(Proverbs 11:17)

 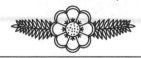

DAY 19	SU MO TU WE TH FR SA DATE: _____	How Do I Feel Today

BREAKFAST	LUNCH	DINNER

SNACKS:

TOTAL CALORIES	GLASSES OF WATER	HOURS OF SLEEP

WEIGHT	BLOOD PRESSURE	BLOOD SUGAR

EXERCISE/ PHYSICAL ACTIVITY	SELF-CARE ACTIVITY

He restores my soul. He leads me in paths of righteousness for his name's sake.
(Psalm 23:3)

DAY 20

SU MO TU WE TH FR SA

DATE: _____

How Do I Feel Today

BREAKFAST	LUNCH	DINNER

SNACKS:

TOTAL CALORIES	GLASSES OF WATER	HOURS OF SLEEP

WEIGHT	BLOOD PRESSURE	BLOOD SUGAR

EXERCISE/ PHYSICAL ACTIVITY	SELF-CARE ACTIVITY

DAY 21	SU MO TU WE TH FR SA DATE: _____	How Do I Feel Today

BREAKFAST	LUNCH	DINNER

SNACKS:

TOTAL CALORIES	GLASSES OF WATER	HOURS OF SLEEP

WEIGHT	BLOOD PRESSURE	BLOOD SUGAR

EXERCISE/ PHYSICAL ACTIVITY	SELF-CARE ACTIVITY

The Lord will guide me continually and satisfy my desire in scorched places and make my bones strong.
(Isaiah 58:11)

DAY 22	SU MO TU WE TH FR SA DATE: _____	How Do I Feel Today

BREAKFAST	LUNCH	DINNER

SNACKS:

TOTAL CALORIES	GLASSES OF WATER	HOURS OF SLEEP

WEIGHT	BLOOD PRESSURE	BLOOD SUGAR

EXERCISE/ PHYSICAL ACTIVITY	SELF-CARE ACTIVITY

I am like a well-watered garden, like a spring whose waters never fail.
(Isaiah 58:11)

 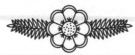

DAY 23	SU MO TU WE TH FR SA DATE: _____	How Do I Feel Today

BREAKFAST	LUNCH	DINNER

SNACKS:

TOTAL CALORIES	GLASSES OF WATER	HOURS OF SLEEP

WEIGHT	BLOOD PRESSURE	BLOOD SUGAR

EXERCISE/ PHYSICAL ACTIVITY	SELF-CARE ACTIVITY

I will be anxious for nothing, but with prayer and petition, with thanksgiving, I will present my requests to God, and the peace of God, which surpasses all understanding, will guard my heart and mind in Christ Jesus.
(Philippians 4:7)

 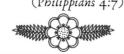

DAY 24

SU MO TU WE TH FR SA

DATE: _____

How Do I Feel Today

☐ ☐ ☐ ☐

BREAKFAST	LUNCH	DINNER

SNACKS:

TOTAL CALORIES	GLASSES OF WATER	HOURS OF SLEEP

WEIGHT	BLOOD PRESSURE	BLOOD SUGAR

EXERCISE/ PHYSICAL ACTIVITY	SELF-CARE ACTIVITY

You will keep me in perfect peace because my mind is stayed on you, and I trust in you, oh Lord.
(Isaiah 26:3)

 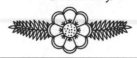

DAY 25	SU MO TU WE TH FR SA DATE: _____	How Do I Feel Today

BREAKFAST	LUNCH	DINNER

SNACKS:

TOTAL CALORIES	GLASSES OF WATER	HOURS OF SLEEP

WEIGHT	BLOOD PRESSURE	BLOOD SUGAR

EXERCISE/ PHYSICAL ACTIVITY	SELF-CARE ACTIVITY

I will pay close attention to my life and your teachings, oh Lord; I will persevere in all things, for in so doing I will save both myself and my hearers. (1 Timothy 4:16)

 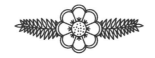

DAY 26

SU MO TU WE TH FR SA

DATE: _____

How Do I Feel Today

BREAKFAST	LUNCH	DINNER

SNACKS:

TOTAL CALORIES	GLASSES OF WATER	HOURS OF SLEEP

WEIGHT	BLOOD PRESSURE	BLOOD SUGAR

EXERCISE/ PHYSICAL ACTIVITY	SELF-CARE ACTIVITY

*I will practice your teaching, oh Lords; I will be committed to them,
so that my progress will be evident to all.* (1 Timothy 4:15)

 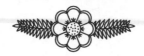

DAY 27

SU MO TU WE TH FR SA

DATE: _____

How Do I Feel Today

BREAKFAST	LUNCH	DINNER

SNACKS:

TOTAL CALORIES	GLASSES OF WATER	HOURS OF SLEEP

WEIGHT	BLOOD PRESSURE	BLOOD SUGAR

EXERCISE/ PHYSICAL ACTIVITY	SELF-CARE ACTIVITY

I discipline my body and keep it under control, so that after preaching to others,
I myself will not be disqualified. (1 Corinthians 9:27)

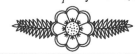

DAY 28	SU MO TU WE TH FR SA DATE: _____	How Do I Feel Today

BREAKFAST	LUNCH	DINNER

SNACKS:

TOTAL CALORIES	GLASSES OF WATER	HOURS OF SLEEP

WEIGHT	BLOOD PRESSURE	BLOOD SUGAR

EXERCISE/ PHYSICAL ACTIVITY	SELF-CARE ACTIVITY

I will love the Lord my God with all my heart and with all my soul and with all my mind.
(Matthew 22:37)

DAY 29

SU MO TU WE TH FR SA

DATE: _____

How Do I Feel Today

BREAKFAST	LUNCH	DINNER

SNACKS:

TOTAL CALORIES	GLASSES OF WATER	HOURS OF SLEEP

WEIGHT	BLOOD PRESSURE	BLOOD SUGAR

EXERCISE/ PHYSICAL ACTIVITY	SELF-CARE ACTIVITY

Whatever is true, whatever is honorable, whatever is just, whatever is pure, whatever is lovely, whatever is commendable, if there is any excellence, if there is anything worthy of praise, I will focus on those things.
(Philippians 4:8)

 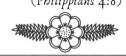

DAY 30	SU MO TU WE TH FR SA DATE: _____	How Do I Feel Today

BREAKFAST	LUNCH	DINNER

SNACKS:

TOTAL CALORIES	GLASSES OF WATER	HOURS OF SLEEP

WEIGHT	BLOOD PRESSURE	BLOOD SUGAR

EXERCISE/ PHYSICAL ACTIVITY	SELF-CARE ACTIVITY

I will seek the Lord, when I feel weary and burdened, and He will give me rest.
(Matthew 11:28)

DAY 31	SU MO TU WE TH FR SA DATE: _____	How Do I Feel Today 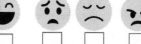

BREAKFAST	LUNCH	DINNER

SNACKS:

TOTAL CALORIES	GLASSES OF WATER	HOURS OF SLEEP

WEIGHT	BLOOD PRESSURE	BLOOD SUGAR

EXERCISE/ PHYSICAL ACTIVITY	SELF-CARE ACTIVITY

I will trust in the Lord with my whole heart and never rely on what I think I know.
(Proverbs 3:5)

DAY 32	SU MO TU WE TH FR SA DATE: _____	How Do I Feel Today

BREAKFAST	LUNCH	DINNER

SNACKS:

TOTAL CALORIES	GLASSES OF WATER	HOURS OF SLEEP

WEIGHT	BLOOD PRESSURE	BLOOD SUGAR

EXERCISE/ PHYSICAL ACTIVITY	SELF-CARE ACTIVITY

I will always allow the Lord to lead me, and he will show me the right path to take.
(Proverbs 3:6)

 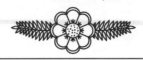

DAY 33

SU MO TU WE TH FR SA

DATE: _____

How Do I Feel Today

BREAKFAST	LUNCH	DINNER

SNACKS:

TOTAL CALORIES	GLASSES OF WATER	HOURS OF SLEEP

WEIGHT	BLOOD PRESSURE	BLOOD SUGAR

EXERCISE/ PHYSICAL ACTIVITY	SELF-CARE ACTIVITY

You are my hiding place, oh Lord; you will protect me from trouble and surround me with songs of deliverance. (Psalm 32:7-8)

 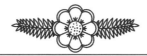

DAY 34	SU MO TU WE TH FR SA DATE: _____	How Do I Feel Today

BREAKFAST	LUNCH	DINNER

SNACKS:

TOTAL CALORIES	GLASSES OF WATER	HOURS OF SLEEP

WEIGHT	BLOOD PRESSURE	BLOOD SUGAR

EXERCISE/ PHYSICAL ACTIVITY	SELF-CARE ACTIVITY

I am chosen and loved by God. (Colossians 3:12)

 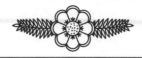

DAY 35	SU MO TU WE TH FR SA DATE: _____	How Do I Feel Today

BREAKFAST	LUNCH	DINNER

SNACKS:

TOTAL CALORIES	GLASSES OF WATER	HOURS OF SLEEP

WEIGHT	BLOOD PRESSURE	BLOOD SUGAR

EXERCISE/ PHYSICAL ACTIVITY	SELF-CARE ACTIVITY

My God will supply all of my needs according to his riches in glory, in Christ Jesus.
(Philippians 4:19)

DAY 36

SU MO TU WE TH FR SA

DATE: _____

How Do I Feel Today

BREAKFAST	LUNCH	DINNER

SNACKS:

TOTAL CALORIES	GLASSES OF WATER	HOURS OF SLEEP

WEIGHT	BLOOD PRESSURE	BLOOD SUGAR

EXERCISE/ PHYSICAL ACTIVITY	SELF-CARE ACTIVITY

I will have complete boldness, so that now as always, Christ will be honored in my body.
(Philippians 1:20)

DAY 37

SU MO TU WE TH FR SA

DATE: _____

How Do I Feel Today

☐ ☐ ☐ ☐

BREAKFAST	LUNCH	DINNER

SNACKS:

TOTAL CALORIES	GLASSES OF WATER	HOURS OF SLEEP

WEIGHT	BLOOD PRESSURE	BLOOD SUGAR

EXERCISE/ PHYSICAL ACTIVITY	SELF-CARE ACTIVITY

For no one ever hated his own flesh, but nourishes and cherishes it, just as Christ does the church, because I am a member of his body. (Ephesians 5:29-30)

DAY 38

SU MO TU WE TH FR SA

DATE: _____

How Do I Feel Today

BREAKFAST	LUNCH	DINNER

SNACKS:

TOTAL CALORIES	GLASSES OF WATER	HOURS OF SLEEP

WEIGHT	BLOOD PRESSURE	BLOOD SUGAR

EXERCISE/ PHYSICAL ACTIVITY	SELF-CARE ACTIVITY

The eye is the lamp of the body. So, if my eye is healthy, my whole body will be full of light
(Matthew 6:22)

 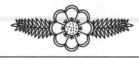

DAY 39

SU MO TU WE TH FR SA

DATE: _____

How Do I Feel Today

BREAKFAST	LUNCH	DINNER

SNACKS:

TOTAL CALORIES	GLASSES OF WATER	HOURS OF SLEEP

WEIGHT	BLOOD PRESSURE	BLOOD SUGAR

EXERCISE/ PHYSICAL ACTIVITY	SELF-CARE ACTIVITY

It is not for kings to drink wine, or for rulers to take strong drink, lest they drink and forget what has been decreed and pervert the rights of all the afflicted. (Proverbs 31:4-5)

 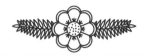

DAY 40	SU MO TU WE TH FR SA DATE: _____	How Do I Feel Today

BREAKFAST	LUNCH	DINNER

SNACKS:

TOTAL CALORIES	GLASSES OF WATER	HOURS OF SLEEP

WEIGHT	BLOOD PRESSURE	BLOOD SUGAR

EXERCISE/ PHYSICAL ACTIVITY	SELF-CARE ACTIVITY

For you formed my inward parts, oh Lord; you knitted me together in my mother's womb.
(Psalm 139:13)

DAY 41

SU MO TU WE TH FR SA

DATE: _____

How Do I Feel Today

BREAKFAST	LUNCH	DINNER

SNACKS:

TOTAL CALORIES	GLASSES OF WATER	HOURS OF SLEEP

WEIGHT	BLOOD PRESSURE	BLOOD SUGAR

EXERCISE/ PHYSICAL ACTIVITY	SELF-CARE ACTIVITY

I will lay aside every weight, and sin, which tries to cling so closely to me.
(Hebrews 12:1)

DAY 42	SU MO TU WE TH FR SA DATE: _____	How Do I Feel Today

BREAKFAST	LUNCH	DINNER

SNACKS:

TOTAL CALORIES	GLASSES OF WATER	HOURS OF SLEEP

WEIGHT	BLOOD PRESSURE	BLOOD SUGAR

EXERCISE/ PHYSICAL ACTIVITY	SELF-CARE ACTIVITY

I will fix my eyes on Jesus, the founder and perfecter of my faith.
(Hebrews 12: 2)

 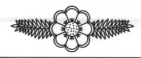

DAY 43	SU MO TU WE TH FR SA	How Do I Feel Today
	DATE: ————————	

BREAKFAST	LUNCH	DINNER

SNACKS:

TOTAL CALORIES	GLASSES OF WATER	HOURS OF SLEEP

WEIGHT	BLOOD PRESSURE	BLOOD SUGAR

EXERCISE/ PHYSICAL ACTIVITY	SELF-CARE ACTIVITY

When the righteous cry for help, the Lord hears, and rescues them from all their troubles.
(Psalm 34:17)

 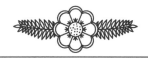

DAY 44

SU MO TU WE TH FR SA

DATE: _____

How Do I Feel Today

BREAKFAST	LUNCH	DINNER

SNACKS:

TOTAL CALORIES	GLASSES OF WATER	HOURS OF SLEEP

WEIGHT	BLOOD PRESSURE	BLOOD SUGAR

EXERCISE/ PHYSICAL ACTIVITY	SELF-CARE ACTIVITY

I was bought with a price. Therefore, I will glorify God with my body.
(1 *Corinthians* 6:20)

 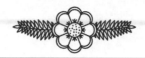

DAY 45	SU MO TU WE TH FR SA DATE: _____	How Do I Feel Today

BREAKFAST	LUNCH	DINNER

SNACKS:

TOTAL CALORIES	GLASSES OF WATER	HOURS OF SLEEP

WEIGHT	BLOOD PRESSURE	BLOOD SUGAR

EXERCISE/ PHYSICAL ACTIVITY	SELF-CARE ACTIVITY

Peace of mind makes the body healthy; but envy rots the bones.
(Proverbs 14:30)

 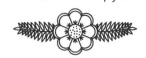

DAY 46	SU MO TU WE TH FR SA DATE: _____	How Do I Feel Today

BREAKFAST	LUNCH	DINNER

SNACKS:

TOTAL CALORIES	GLASSES OF WATER	HOURS OF SLEEP

WEIGHT	BLOOD PRESSURE	BLOOD SUGAR

EXERCISE/ PHYSICAL ACTIVITY	SELF-CARE ACTIVITY

I will show love for others by truly helping them, and not merely talk about it.
(1 John 3:18)

 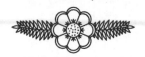

DAY 47	SU MO TU WE TH FR SA DATE: _____	How Do I Feel Today

BREAKFAST	LUNCH	DINNER

SNACKS:

TOTAL CALORIES	GLASSES OF WATER	HOURS OF SLEEP

WEIGHT	BLOOD PRESSURE	BLOOD SUGAR

EXERCISE/ PHYSICAL ACTIVITY	SELF-CARE ACTIVITY

For God gave me a spirit, not of fear, but of power and love and self-control.
(2 Timothy 1:7)

DAY 48	SU MO TU WE TH FR SA DATE: _____	How Do I Feel Today ☐ ☐ ☐ ☐

BREAKFAST	LUNCH	DINNER

SNACKS:

TOTAL CALORIES	GLASSES OF WATER	HOURS OF SLEEP

WEIGHT	BLOOD PRESSURE	BLOOD SUGAR

EXERCISE/ PHYSICAL ACTIVITY	SELF-CARE ACTIVITY

I will be happy in the Lord, and he will give me my heart's desire.
(Psalm 37:4)

DAY 49	SU MO TU WE TH FR SA DATE: _____	How Do I Feel Today

BREAKFAST	LUNCH	DINNER

SNACKS:

TOTAL CALORIES	GLASSES OF WATER	HOURS OF SLEEP

WEIGHT	BLOOD PRESSURE	BLOOD SUGAR

EXERCISE/ PHYSICAL ACTIVITY	SELF-CARE ACTIVITY

Man shall not live by bread alone, but by every word that comes from the mouth of God.
(Matthew 4:4)

DAY 50	SU MO TU WE TH FR SA DATE: _____	How Do I Feel Today

BREAKFAST	LUNCH	DINNER

SNACKS:

TOTAL CALORIES	GLASSES OF WATER	HOURS OF SLEEP

WEIGHT	BLOOD PRESSURE	BLOOD SUGAR

EXERCISE/ PHYSICAL ACTIVITY	SELF-CARE ACTIVITY

The Lord is near to all who call on him. He fulfills the desires of those who fear him; he hears their cry and saves them. (Psalm 145: 18-19)

 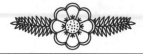

DAY 51	SU MO TU WE TH FR SA	How Do I Feel Today
	DATE: _____	☐ ☐ ☐ ☐

BREAKFAST	LUNCH	DINNER

SNACKS:

TOTAL CALORIES	GLASSES OF WATER	HOURS OF SLEEP

WEIGHT	BLOOD PRESSURE	BLOOD SUGAR

EXERCISE/ PHYSICAL ACTIVITY	SELF-CARE ACTIVITY

I was made in the image and likeness of God.
(Genesis 1:26)

DAY 52

SU MO TU WE TH FR SA

DATE: _____

How Do I Feel Today

BREAKFAST	LUNCH	DINNER

SNACKS:

TOTAL CALORIES	GLASSES OF WATER	HOURS OF SLEEP

WEIGHT	BLOOD PRESSURE	BLOOD SUGAR

EXERCISE/ PHYSICAL ACTIVITY	SELF-CARE ACTIVITY

I was made to have dominion over all the Earth and over every living thing that creeps on the earth.
(Genesis 1:26)

DAY 53

SU MO TU WE TH FR SA

DATE: _____

How Do I Feel Today

☐	☐	☐	☐

BREAKFAST	LUNCH	DINNER

SNACKS:

TOTAL CALORIES	GLASSES OF WATER	HOURS OF SLEEP

WEIGHT	BLOOD PRESSURE	BLOOD SUGAR

EXERCISE/ PHYSICAL ACTIVITY	SELF-CARE ACTIVITY

From Him my whole body is fitted and held together by every supporting ligament; and as each individual part does its work, my body will grow and build itself up in love. (Ephesians 4:16)

 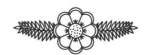

DAY 54	SU MO TU WE TH FR SA DATE: _____	How Do I Feel Today ☐ ☐ ☐ ☐

BREAKFAST	LUNCH	DINNER

SNACKS:

TOTAL CALORIES	GLASSES OF WATER	HOURS OF SLEEP

WEIGHT	BLOOD PRESSURE	BLOOD SUGAR

EXERCISE/ PHYSICAL ACTIVITY	SELF-CARE ACTIVITY

I will grow to become in every respect the mature body of Christ, who is the head of my life.
(Ephesians 4:15)

DAY 55	SU MO TU WE TH FR SA DATE: _____	How Do I Feel Today

BREAKFAST	LUNCH	DINNER

SNACKS:

TOTAL CALORIES	GLASSES OF WATER	HOURS OF SLEEP

WEIGHT	BLOOD PRESSURE	BLOOD SUGAR

EXERCISE/ PHYSICAL ACTIVITY	SELF-CARE ACTIVITY

Jesus came, so that I will have life and have it more abundantly.
(John 10:10)

DAY 56	SU MO TU WE TH FR SA DATE: _____	How Do I Feel Today

BREAKFAST	LUNCH	DINNER

SNACKS:

TOTAL CALORIES	GLASSES OF WATER	HOURS OF SLEEP

WEIGHT	BLOOD PRESSURE	BLOOD SUGAR

EXERCISE/ PHYSICAL ACTIVITY	SELF-CARE ACTIVITY

Daniel resolved that he would not defile himself with the king's food, or with the wine that he drank.
(Daniel 1:8)

 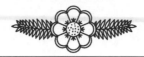

DAY 57	SU MO TU WE TH FR SA DATE: _____	How Do I Feel Today

BREAKFAST	LUNCH	DINNER

SNACKS:

TOTAL CALORIES	GLASSES OF WATER	HOURS OF SLEEP

WEIGHT	BLOOD PRESSURE	BLOOD SUGAR

EXERCISE/ PHYSICAL ACTIVITY	SELF-CARE ACTIVITY

For God is working in me, giving me the desire and the power to do what pleases him.
(Philippians 2:13)

DAY 58	SU MO TU WE TH FR SA DATE: _____	How Do I Feel Today ☐ ☐ ☐ ☐

BREAKFAST	LUNCH	DINNER

SNACKS:

TOTAL CALORIES	GLASSES OF WATER	HOURS OF SLEEP

WEIGHT	BLOOD PRESSURE	BLOOD SUGAR

EXERCISE/ PHYSICAL ACTIVITY	SELF-CARE ACTIVITY

I will approach the throne of grace with boldness, so that I will receive mercy and find grace to help me in times of need. (Hebrews 4:16)

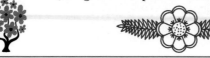

DAY 59	SU MO TU WE TH FR SA DATE: _____	How Do I Feel Today ☐ ☐ ☐ ☐

BREAKFAST	LUNCH	DINNER

SNACKS:

TOTAL CALORIES	GLASSES OF WATER	HOURS OF SLEEP

WEIGHT	BLOOD PRESSURE	BLOOD SUGAR

EXERCISE/ PHYSICAL ACTIVITY	SELF-CARE ACTIVITY

The earnest prayer of a righteous person is powerful and effective.
(James 5:16)

DAY 60	SU MO TU WE TH FR SA DATE: _____	How Do I Feel Today

BREAKFAST	LUNCH	DINNER

SNACKS:

TOTAL CALORIES	GLASSES OF WATER	HOURS OF SLEEP

WEIGHT	BLOOD PRESSURE	BLOOD SUGAR

EXERCISE/ PHYSICAL ACTIVITY	SELF-CARE ACTIVITY

With God all things are possible. (Luke 1:37)

 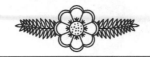

DAY 61	SU MO TU WE TH FR SA	How Do I Feel Today
	DATE: _____	

BREAKFAST	LUNCH	DINNER

SNACKS:

TOTAL CALORIES	GLASSES OF WATER	HOURS OF SLEEP

WEIGHT	BLOOD PRESSURE	BLOOD SUGAR

EXERCISE/ PHYSICAL ACTIVITY	SELF-CARE ACTIVITY

I will put away, anger, wrath, malice, slander, and obscene talk from your mouth.
(Colossians 3:8)

DAY 62	SU MO TU WE TH FR SA DATE: _____	How Do I Feel Today

BREAKFAST	LUNCH	DINNER

SNACKS:

TOTAL CALORIES	GLASSES OF WATER	HOURS OF SLEEP

WEIGHT	BLOOD PRESSURE	BLOOD SUGAR

EXERCISE/ PHYSICAL ACTIVITY	SELF-CARE ACTIVITY

In all labor there is profit, But mere talk leads only to poverty.
(Proverbs 14:23)

DAY 63	SU MO TU WE TH FR SA DATE: _____	How Do I Feel Today

BREAKFAST	LUNCH	DINNER

SNACKS:

TOTAL CALORIES	GLASSES OF WATER	HOURS OF SLEEP

WEIGHT	BLOOD PRESSURE	BLOOD SUGAR

EXERCISE/ PHYSICAL ACTIVITY	SELF-CARE ACTIVITY

The Lord will help me and rescue me; he will deliver me from all evil, because, I seek his protection.
(Psalm 37:40)

DAY 64	SU MO TU WE TH FR SA DATE: _____	How Do I Feel Today

BREAKFAST	LUNCH	DINNER

SNACKS:

TOTAL CALORIES	GLASSES OF WATER	HOURS OF SLEEP

WEIGHT	BLOOD PRESSURE	BLOOD SUGAR

EXERCISE/ PHYSICAL ACTIVITY	SELF-CARE ACTIVITY

The Lord rescues the godly; he is my stronghold in times of trouble.
(Psalms 37:39)

DAY 65

SU MO TU WE TH FR SA

DATE: _____

How Do I Feel Today

BREAKFAST	LUNCH	DINNER

SNACKS:

TOTAL CALORIES	GLASSES OF WATER	HOURS OF SLEEP

WEIGHT	BLOOD PRESSURE	BLOOD SUGAR

EXERCISE/ PHYSICAL ACTIVITY	SELF-CARE ACTIVITY

A great future awaits those who love peace. (Psalm 37:37)

 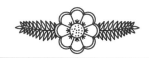

DAY 66	SU MO TU WE TH FR SA DATE: _____	How Do I Feel Today

BREAKFAST	LUNCH	DINNER

SNACKS:

TOTAL CALORIES	GLASSES OF WATER	HOURS OF SLEEP

WEIGHT	BLOOD PRESSURE	BLOOD SUGAR

EXERCISE/ PHYSICAL ACTIVITY	SELF-CARE ACTIVITY

The word of God is alive and powerful! It is sharper than any double-edged sword.
(Hebrews 4:12)

 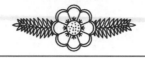

DAY 67	SU MO TU WE TH FR SA DATE: _____	How Do I Feel Today

BREAKFAST	LUNCH	DINNER

SNACKS:

TOTAL CALORIES	GLASSES OF WATER	HOURS OF SLEEP

WEIGHT	BLOOD PRESSURE	BLOOD SUGAR

EXERCISE/ PHYSICAL ACTIVITY	SELF-CARE ACTIVITY

Lord, you alone deserves all of the praise, because of your love and faithfulness.
(Psalm 115:1)

 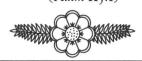

DAY 68	SU MO TU WE TH FR SA DATE: _____	How Do I Feel Today

BREAKFAST	LUNCH	DINNER

SNACKS:

TOTAL CALORIES	GLASSES OF WATER	HOURS OF SLEEP

WEIGHT	BLOOD PRESSURE	BLOOD SUGAR

EXERCISE/ PHYSICAL ACTIVITY	SELF-CARE ACTIVITY

I will extol the Lord, both now and forevermore. Praise the Lord!
(Psalm 115:18)

DAY 69	SU MO TU WE TH FR SA DATE: _____	How Do I Feel Today ☐ ☐ ☐ ☐

BREAKFAST	LUNCH	DINNER

SNACKS:

TOTAL CALORIES	GLASSES OF WATER	HOURS OF SLEEP

WEIGHT	BLOOD PRESSURE	BLOOD SUGAR

EXERCISE/ PHYSICAL ACTIVITY	SELF-CARE ACTIVITY

I am blessed by the Lord, the Maker of Heaven and Earth. (Psalm 115:15)

DAY 70	SU MO TU WE TH FR SA DATE: _____	How Do I Feel Today

BREAKFAST	LUNCH	DINNER

SNACKS:

TOTAL CALORIES	GLASSES OF WATER	HOURS OF SLEEP

WEIGHT	BLOOD PRESSURE	BLOOD SUGAR

EXERCISE/ PHYSICAL ACTIVITY	SELF-CARE ACTIVITY

He will not allow any disease to overtake me, for He is the Lord, my healer.
(Exodus 15:26)

| DAY 71 | SU MO TU WE TH FR SA
DATE: _____ | How Do I Feel Today |

BREAKFAST	LUNCH	DINNER

SNACKS:

TOTAL CALORIES	GLASSES OF WATER	HOURS OF SLEEP

WEIGHT	BLOOD PRESSURE	BLOOD SUGAR

EXERCISE/ PHYSICAL ACTIVITY	SELF-CARE ACTIVITY

His blessing will be on my food and water and He will take away sickness from me.
(Exodus 23:25)

 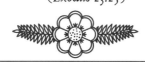

DAY 72	SU MO TU WE TH FR SA DATE: _____	How Do I Feel Today

BREAKFAST	LUNCH	DINNER

SNACKS:

TOTAL CALORIES	GLASSES OF WATER	HOURS OF SLEEP

WEIGHT	BLOOD PRESSURE	BLOOD SUGAR

EXERCISE/ PHYSICAL ACTIVITY	SELF-CARE ACTIVITY

I will not fear for God is with you; I will not be dismayed, for He is my God.
He will strengthen me and help me; He will uphold me with His righteous right hand.
(Isaiah 41:10)

DAY 73	SU MO TU WE TH FR SA	How Do I Feel Today
	DATE: _____	

BREAKFAST	LUNCH	DINNER

SNACKS:

TOTAL CALORIES	GLASSES OF WATER	HOURS OF SLEEP

WEIGHT	BLOOD PRESSURE	BLOOD SUGAR

EXERCISE/ PHYSICAL ACTIVITY	SELF-CARE ACTIVITY

By His wounds I am healed.
(Isaiah 53:5)

 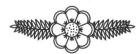

DAY 74	SU MO TU WE TH FR SA DATE: _____	How Do I Feel Today

BREAKFAST	LUNCH	DINNER

SNACKS:

TOTAL CALORIES	GLASSES OF WATER	HOURS OF SLEEP

WEIGHT	BLOOD PRESSURE	BLOOD SUGAR

EXERCISE/ PHYSICAL ACTIVITY	SELF-CARE ACTIVITY

He gives strength to the weary and increases the power of the weak.
(Isaiah 40:29)

 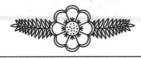

DAY 75	SU MO TU WE TH FR SA DATE: _____	How Do I Feel Today

BREAKFAST	LUNCH	DINNER

SNACKS:

TOTAL CALORIES	GLASSES OF WATER	HOURS OF SLEEP

WEIGHT	BLOOD PRESSURE	BLOOD SUGAR

EXERCISE/ PHYSICAL ACTIVITY	SELF-CARE ACTIVITY

When I am tempted, He will provide a way out, so that, I will be able to endure it.
(1 Corinthians 10:13)

 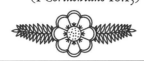

DAY 76

SU MO TU WE TH FR SA

DATE: _____

How Do I Feel Today

☐ ☐ ☐ ☐

BREAKFAST	LUNCH	DINNER

SNACKS:

TOTAL CALORIES	GLASSES OF WATER	HOURS OF SLEEP

WEIGHT	BLOOD PRESSURE	BLOOD SUGAR

EXERCISE/ PHYSICAL ACTIVITY	SELF-CARE ACTIVITY

The Lord redeems my life from the pit and crowns me with love and compassion.
(Psalms 103:4)

DAY 77

SU MO TU WE TH FR SA

DATE: _____

How Do I Feel Today

☐ ☐ ☐ ☐

BREAKFAST	LUNCH	DINNER

SNACKS:

TOTAL CALORIES	GLASSES OF WATER	HOURS OF SLEEP

WEIGHT	BLOOD PRESSURE	BLOOD SUGAR

EXERCISE/ PHYSICAL ACTIVITY	SELF-CARE ACTIVITY

My heart rejoices in Your salvation, oh Lord. (Psalm 13:5)

 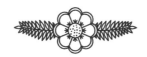

DAY 78	SU MO TU WE TH FR SA DATE: _____	How Do I Feel Today

BREAKFAST	LUNCH	DINNER

SNACKS:

TOTAL CALORIES	GLASSES OF WATER	HOURS OF SLEEP

WEIGHT	BLOOD PRESSURE	BLOOD SUGAR

EXERCISE/ PHYSICAL ACTIVITY	SELF-CARE ACTIVITY

I trust in your unfailing love, oh Lord. (Psalm 13:5)

 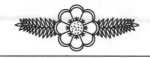

DAY 79

SU MO TU WE TH FR SA

DATE: _____

How Do I Feel Today

BREAKFAST	LUNCH	DINNER

SNACKS:

TOTAL CALORIES	GLASSES OF WATER	HOURS OF SLEEP

WEIGHT	BLOOD PRESSURE	BLOOD SUGAR

EXERCISE/ PHYSICAL ACTIVITY	SELF-CARE ACTIVITY

He will satisfy me with a long life, And show me His salvation.   (Psalm 91:16)

 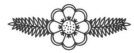

DAY 80

SU MO TU WE TH FR SA

DATE: _____

How Do I Feel Today

BREAKFAST	LUNCH	DINNER

SNACKS:

TOTAL CALORIES	GLASSES OF WATER	HOURS OF SLEEP

WEIGHT	BLOOD PRESSURE	BLOOD SUGAR

EXERCISE/ PHYSICAL ACTIVITY	SELF-CARE ACTIVITY

The Lord is my strength and song, And He has become my salvation.
(Psalm 118:14)

 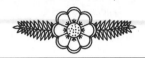

| DAY 81 | SU MO TU WE TH FR SA

DATE: _____ | How Do I Feel Today |

BREAKFAST	LUNCH	DINNER

SNACKS:

TOTAL CALORIES	GLASSES OF WATER	HOURS OF SLEEP

WEIGHT	BLOOD PRESSURE	BLOOD SUGAR

EXERCISE/ PHYSICAL ACTIVITY	SELF-CARE ACTIVITY

God is my salvation, I will trust in Him and not be afraid. (Isaiah 12:2)

| DAY 82 | SU MO TU WE TH FR SA

DATE: _____ | How Do I Feel Today |
|---|---|---|

BREAKFAST	LUNCH	DINNER

SNACKS:

TOTAL CALORIES	GLASSES OF WATER	HOURS OF SLEEP

WEIGHT	BLOOD PRESSURE	BLOOD SUGAR

EXERCISE/ PHYSICAL ACTIVITY	SELF-CARE ACTIVITY

The Lord himself, is my strength and my defense. He will always come to my rescue.
(Isaiah 12:2)

 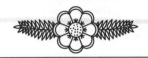

DAY 83	SU MO TU WE TH FR SA DATE: _____	How Do I Feel Today

BREAKFAST	LUNCH	DINNER

SNACKS:

TOTAL CALORIES	GLASSES OF WATER	HOURS OF SLEEP

WEIGHT	BLOOD PRESSURE	BLOOD SUGAR

EXERCISE/ PHYSICAL ACTIVITY	SELF-CARE ACTIVITY

The Lord will sanctify me completely. He will preserve my spirit, soul and body.
(1 Thessalonian 5:23)

DAY 84	SU MO TU WE TH FR SA DATE: _____	How Do I Feel Today

BREAKFAST	LUNCH	DINNER

SNACKS:

TOTAL CALORIES	GLASSES OF WATER	HOURS OF SLEEP

WEIGHT	BLOOD PRESSURE	BLOOD SUGAR

EXERCISE/ PHYSICAL ACTIVITY	SELF-CARE ACTIVITY

I will have a long life; His peace will be upon me, upon my family, and upon all my possessions.
(1 Samuel 25:6)

DAY 85

SU MO TU WE TH FR SA

DATE: _____

How Do I Feel Today

BREAKFAST	LUNCH	DINNER

SNACKS:

TOTAL CALORIES	GLASSES OF WATER	HOURS OF SLEEP

WEIGHT	BLOOD PRESSURE	BLOOD SUGAR

EXERCISE/ PHYSICAL ACTIVITY	SELF-CARE ACTIVITY

The Lord will bring health and healing to my body, and will reveal to me an abundance of peace and truth. (Jeremiah 33:6)

 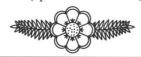

DAY 86	SU MO TU WE TH FR SA DATE: _____	How Do I Feel Today ☺ 😟 😣 😠 ☐ ☐ ☐ ☐

BREAKFAST	LUNCH	DINNER

SNACKS:

TOTAL CALORIES	GLASSES OF WATER	HOURS OF SLEEP

WEIGHT	BLOOD PRESSURE	BLOOD SUGAR

EXERCISE/ PHYSICAL ACTIVITY	SELF-CARE ACTIVITY

I will keep His words in the midst of my heart. For they will give life and good health to my body.
(Proverbs 4:20 - 22)

 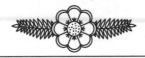

DAY 87	SU MO TU WE TH FR SA	How Do I Feel Today
	DATE: _____	☐ ☐ ☐ ☐

BREAKFAST	LUNCH	DINNER

SNACKS:

TOTAL CALORIES	GLASSES OF WATER	HOURS OF SLEEP

WEIGHT	BLOOD PRESSURE	BLOOD SUGAR

EXERCISE/ PHYSICAL ACTIVITY	SELF-CARE ACTIVITY

Godliness is profitable for all things, since it holds promise
for the present life and also for the life to come. (1 Timothy 4:8)

 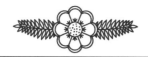

DAY 88	SU MO TU WE TH FR SA DATE: _____	How Do I Feel Today ☐ ☐ ☐ ☐

BREAKFAST	LUNCH	DINNER

SNACKS:

TOTAL CALORIES	GLASSES OF WATER	HOURS OF SLEEP

WEIGHT	BLOOD PRESSURE	BLOOD SUGAR

EXERCISE/ PHYSICAL ACTIVITY	SELF-CARE ACTIVITY

The steadfast love of the LORD never ceases; his mercies never come to an end;
they are new every morning; great is His faithfulness.   (Lamentations 3:22-23:)

 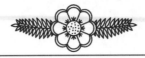

DAY 89

SU MO TU WE TH FR SA

DATE: _____

How Do I Feel Today

BREAKFAST	LUNCH	DINNER

SNACKS:

TOTAL CALORIES	GLASSES OF WATER	HOURS OF SLEEP

WEIGHT	BLOOD PRESSURE	BLOOD SUGAR

EXERCISE/ PHYSICAL ACTIVITY	SELF-CARE ACTIVITY

The name of the LORD is a strong tower; the righteous runs into it and is safe.
(Proverbs 18:10)

DAY 90

SU MO TU WE TH FR SA

DATE: ———————————

How Do I Feel Today

BREAKFAST	LUNCH	DINNER

SNACKS:

TOTAL CALORIES	GLASSES OF WATER	HOURS OF SLEEP

WEIGHT	BLOOD PRESSURE	BLOOD SUGAR

EXERCISE/ PHYSICAL ACTIVITY	SELF-CARE ACTIVITY

The Lord lives! Praise to my Rock! May God, the Rock of my salvation, be exalted!
(2 Samuel 22:47)

 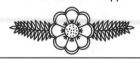

DAY 91	SU MO TU WE TH FR SA DATE: _____	How Do I Feel Today

BREAKFAST	LUNCH	DINNER

SNACKS:

TOTAL CALORIES	GLASSES OF WATER	HOURS OF SLEEP

WEIGHT	BLOOD PRESSURE	BLOOD SUGAR

EXERCISE/ PHYSICAL ACTIVITY	SELF-CARE ACTIVITY

The Lord almighty is with me; the God of Jacob is my fortress.
(Psalm 46:7)

 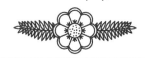

DAY 92	SU MO TU WE TH FR SA DATE: _____	How Do I Feel Today

BREAKFAST	LUNCH	DINNER

SNACKS:

TOTAL CALORIES	GLASSES OF WATER	HOURS OF SLEEP

WEIGHT	BLOOD PRESSURE	BLOOD SUGAR

EXERCISE/ PHYSICAL ACTIVITY	SELF-CARE ACTIVITY

I will cast my burdens on the Lord, for he will sustain me; he will never let me be defeated.
(Psalm 55:22)

DAY 93

SU MO TU WE TH FR SA

DATE: _____

How Do I Feel Today

BREAKFAST	LUNCH	DINNER

SNACKS:

TOTAL CALORIES	GLASSES OF WATER	HOURS OF SLEEP

WEIGHT	BLOOD PRESSURE	BLOOD SUGAR

EXERCISE/ PHYSICAL ACTIVITY	SELF-CARE ACTIVITY

The Lord is my rock and my salvation, He is my fortress; I shall not be shaken.
(Psalm 62:6)

DAY 94	SU MO TU WE TH FR SA DATE: _____	How Do I Feel Today

BREAKFAST	LUNCH	DINNER

SNACKS:

TOTAL CALORIES	GLASSES OF WATER	HOURS OF SLEEP

WEIGHT	BLOOD PRESSURE	BLOOD SUGAR

EXERCISE/ PHYSICAL ACTIVITY	SELF-CARE ACTIVITY

Lord, You are my refuge and my shield; I have put my hope in your word.
(Psalm 119:114)

 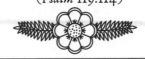

SU MO TU WE TH FR SA

DAY 95

DATE: _____

How Do I Feel Today

☐	☐	☐	☐

BREAKFAST	LUNCH	DINNER

SNACKS:

TOTAL CALORIES	GLASSES OF WATER	HOURS OF SLEEP

WEIGHT	BLOOD PRESSURE	BLOOD SUGAR

EXERCISE/ PHYSICAL ACTIVITY	SELF-CARE ACTIVITY

The Lord is faithful. He will strengthen me and protect me from evil.
(2 Thessalonians 3:3)

 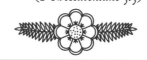

DAY 96	SU MO TU WE TH FR SA DATE: _____	How Do I Feel Today

BREAKFAST	LUNCH	DINNER

SNACKS:

TOTAL CALORIES	GLASSES OF WATER	HOURS OF SLEEP

WEIGHT	BLOOD PRESSURE	BLOOD SUGAR

EXERCISE/ PHYSICAL ACTIVITY	SELF-CARE ACTIVITY

I will go out with joy and be led forth with peace. (Isaiah 55:12)

 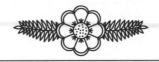

DAY 97

SU MO TU WE TH FR SA

DATE: _____

How Do I Feel Today

☐ ☐ ☐ ☐

BREAKFAST	LUNCH	DINNER

SNACKS:

TOTAL CALORIES	GLASSES OF WATER	HOURS OF SLEEP

WEIGHT	BLOOD PRESSURE	BLOOD SUGAR

EXERCISE/ PHYSICAL ACTIVITY	SELF-CARE ACTIVITY

Surely your goodness and love will follow me all the days of my life. (Psalm 23:6)

 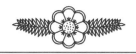

DAY 98	SU MO TU WE TH FR SA DATE: _____	How Do I Feel Today

BREAKFAST	LUNCH	DINNER

SNACKS:

TOTAL CALORIES	GLASSES OF WATER	HOURS OF SLEEP

WEIGHT	BLOOD PRESSURE	BLOOD SUGAR

EXERCISE/ PHYSICAL ACTIVITY	SELF-CARE ACTIVITY

The hope of the righteous brings joy, but the expectation of the wicked will perish.
(Proverbs 10:28)

DAY 99

SU MO TU WE TH FR SA

DATE: _____

How Do I Feel Today

BREAKFAST	LUNCH	DINNER

SNACKS:

TOTAL CALORIES	GLASSES OF WATER	HOURS OF SLEEP

WEIGHT	BLOOD PRESSURE	BLOOD SUGAR

EXERCISE/ PHYSICAL ACTIVITY	SELF-CARE ACTIVITY

I will Rejoice always, pray without ceasing, and give thanks in all circumstances;
For this is the will of God in Christ Jesus for me. (1 Thessalonians 5:16-18)

 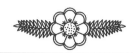

DAY 100

SU MO TU WE TH FR SA

DATE: _____

How Do I Feel Today

BREAKFAST	LUNCH	DINNER

SNACKS:

TOTAL CALORIES	GLASSES OF WATER	HOURS OF SLEEP

WEIGHT	BLOOD PRESSURE	BLOOD SUGAR

EXERCISE/ PHYSICAL ACTIVITY	SELF-CARE ACTIVITY

My heart is glad, my whole being rejoices and my flesh also dwells secure.
(Psalm 16:9)

 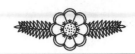

DAY 101

SU MO TU WE TH FR SA

DATE: _____

How Do I Feel Today

BREAKFAST	LUNCH	DINNER

SNACKS:

TOTAL CALORIES	GLASSES OF WATER	HOURS OF SLEEP

WEIGHT	BLOOD PRESSURE	BLOOD SUGAR

EXERCISE/ PHYSICAL ACTIVITY	SELF-CARE ACTIVITY

For his anger is but for a moment, and his favor is for a lifetime. (Psalm 30:5)

 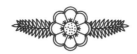

DAY 102	SU MO TU WE TH FR SA DATE: _____	How Do I Feel Today

BREAKFAST	LUNCH	DINNER

SNACKS:

TOTAL CALORIES	GLASSES OF WATER	HOURS OF SLEEP

WEIGHT	BLOOD PRESSURE	BLOOD SUGAR

EXERCISE/ PHYSICAL ACTIVITY	SELF-CARE ACTIVITY

Weeping may tarry for the night, but joy comes with the morning. (Psalm 30:5)

 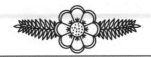 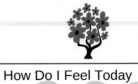

DAY 103	SU MO TU WE TH FR SA DATE: _____	How Do I Feel Today

BREAKFAST	LUNCH	DINNER

SNACKS:

TOTAL CALORIES	GLASSES OF WATER	HOURS OF SLEEP

WEIGHT	BLOOD PRESSURE	BLOOD SUGAR

EXERCISE/ PHYSICAL ACTIVITY	SELF-CARE ACTIVITY

You make known to me the path of life; in your presence there is fullness of joy;
at your right hand are pleasures forevermore.   (Psalm 16:11)

DAY 104	SU MO TU WE TH FR SA DATE: _____	How Do I Feel Today

BREAKFAST	LUNCH	DINNER

SNACKS:

TOTAL CALORIES	GLASSES OF WATER	HOURS OF SLEEP

WEIGHT	BLOOD PRESSURE	BLOOD SUGAR

EXERCISE/ PHYSICAL ACTIVITY	SELF-CARE ACTIVITY

This is the day that the Lord has made; I will rejoice and be glad in it.
(Psalm 118:24)

 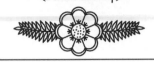

DAY 105

SU MO TU WE TH FR SA

DATE: _____

How Do I Feel Today

☐ ☐ ☐ ☐

BREAKFAST	LUNCH	DINNER

SNACKS:

TOTAL CALORIES	GLASSES OF WATER	HOURS OF SLEEP

WEIGHT	BLOOD PRESSURE	BLOOD SUGAR

EXERCISE/ PHYSICAL ACTIVITY	SELF-CARE ACTIVITY

Send me your light and your faithful care, let them lead me, oh Lord. (Psalm 43:3)

DAY 106	SU MO TU WE TH FR SA DATE: _____	How Do I Feel Today

BREAKFAST	LUNCH	DINNER

SNACKS:

TOTAL CALORIES	GLASSES OF WATER	HOURS OF SLEEP

WEIGHT	BLOOD PRESSURE	BLOOD SUGAR

EXERCISE/ PHYSICAL ACTIVITY	SELF-CARE ACTIVITY

For He shall give His angels charge over me, to keep me in all my ways.   (Psalm 91:11)

 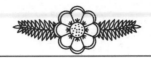

DAY 107

SU MO TU WE TH FR SA

DATE: _____

How Do I Feel Today

BREAKFAST	LUNCH	DINNER

SNACKS:

TOTAL CALORIES	GLASSES OF WATER	HOURS OF SLEEP

WEIGHT	BLOOD PRESSURE	BLOOD SUGAR

EXERCISE/ PHYSICAL ACTIVITY	SELF-CARE ACTIVITY

Whatever I ask for, in the name of Jesus, I will receive, so that my joy may be complete. (John 16:24)

 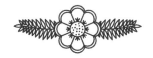

DAY 108

SU MO TU WE TH FR SA

DATE: _____

How Do I Feel Today

BREAKFAST	LUNCH	DINNER

SNACKS:

TOTAL CALORIES	GLASSES OF WATER	HOURS OF SLEEP

WEIGHT	BLOOD PRESSURE	BLOOD SUGAR

EXERCISE/ PHYSICAL ACTIVITY	SELF-CARE ACTIVITY

I possess the fruits of the Spirit: I have love, joy, peace, patience, kindness, goodness, faithfulness, gentleness and self-control. (Galatians 5:22-23)

 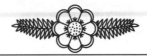

DAY 109

SU MO TU WE TH FR SA

DATE: _____

How Do I Feel Today

BREAKFAST	LUNCH	DINNER

SNACKS:

TOTAL CALORIES	GLASSES OF WATER	HOURS OF SLEEP

WEIGHT	BLOOD PRESSURE	BLOOD SUGAR

EXERCISE/ PHYSICAL ACTIVITY	SELF-CARE ACTIVITY

I will consider it pure joy, whenever I face trials of any kind, because I know that the testing of my faith produces perseverance. (James 1:2-3)

 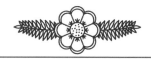

DAY 110	SU MO TU WE TH FR SA DATE: _____	How Do I Feel Today

BREAKFAST	LUNCH	DINNER

SNACKS:

TOTAL CALORIES	GLASSES OF WATER	HOURS OF SLEEP

WEIGHT	BLOOD PRESSURE	BLOOD SUGAR

EXERCISE/ PHYSICAL ACTIVITY	SELF-CARE ACTIVITY

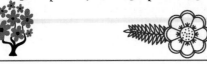

DAY 111	SU MO TU WE TH FR SA DATE: _____	How Do I Feel Today

BREAKFAST	LUNCH	DINNER

SNACKS:

TOTAL CALORIES	GLASSES OF WATER	HOURS OF SLEEP

WEIGHT	BLOOD PRESSURE	BLOOD SUGAR

EXERCISE/ PHYSICAL ACTIVITY	SELF-CARE ACTIVITY

My peace comes from the Lord, so my heart will not be troubled, and I will not be afraid.
(John 14:27)

DAY 112	SU MO TU WE TH FR SA DATE: _____	How Do I Feel Today

BREAKFAST	LUNCH	DINNER

SNACKS:

TOTAL CALORIES	GLASSES OF WATER	HOURS OF SLEEP

WEIGHT	BLOOD PRESSURE	BLOOD SUGAR

EXERCISE/ PHYSICAL ACTIVITY	SELF-CARE ACTIVITY

Splendor and majesty are before the Lord; strength and joy are in his place.
(1 Chronicles 16:27)

DAY 113	SU MO TU WE TH FR SA DATE: _____	How Do I Feel Today

BREAKFAST	LUNCH	DINNER

SNACKS:

TOTAL CALORIES	GLASSES OF WATER	HOURS OF SLEEP

WEIGHT	BLOOD PRESSURE	BLOOD SUGAR

EXERCISE/ PHYSICAL ACTIVITY	SELF-CARE ACTIVITY

You have turned for me my mourning into dancing; you have loosed my sackcloth and clothed me with gladness.   (Psalm 30:11)

 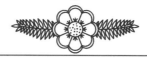

DAY 114	SU MO TU WE TH FR SA DATE: _____	How Do I Feel Today

BREAKFAST	LUNCH	DINNER

SNACKS:

TOTAL CALORIES	GLASSES OF WATER	HOURS OF SLEEP

WEIGHT	BLOOD PRESSURE	BLOOD SUGAR

EXERCISE/ PHYSICAL ACTIVITY	SELF-CARE ACTIVITY

I will look to Jesus, the founder and perfecter of my faith, who for the joy that was set before him endured the cross, despising the shame, and is seated at the right hand of the throne of God.
(Hebrews 12:2)

DAY 115

SU MO TU WE TH FR SA

DATE: _____

How Do I Feel Today

BREAKFAST	LUNCH	DINNER

SNACKS:

TOTAL CALORIES	GLASSES OF WATER	HOURS OF SLEEP

WEIGHT	BLOOD PRESSURE	BLOOD SUGAR

EXERCISE/ PHYSICAL ACTIVITY	SELF-CARE ACTIVITY

All who take refuge in the Lord will rejoice; they will ever sing for joy, because you spread your protection over them, oh Lord; they will rejoice in you. (Psalm 5:11)

DAY 116	SU MO TU WE TH FR SA DATE: _____	How Do I Feel Today

BREAKFAST	LUNCH	DINNER

SNACKS:

TOTAL CALORIES	GLASSES OF WATER	HOURS OF SLEEP

WEIGHT	BLOOD PRESSURE	BLOOD SUGAR

EXERCISE/ PHYSICAL ACTIVITY	SELF-CARE ACTIVITY

I will be strengthened with all power, according to his glorious might,
so that I will have great endurance and patience and joy. (Colossians 1:11)

DAY 117

SU MO TU WE TH FR SA

DATE: _____

How Do I Feel Today

BREAKFAST	LUNCH	DINNER

SNACKS:

TOTAL CALORIES	GLASSES OF WATER	HOURS OF SLEEP

WEIGHT	BLOOD PRESSURE	BLOOD SUGAR

EXERCISE/ PHYSICAL ACTIVITY	SELF-CARE ACTIVITY

For I walk by faith, not by sight.
(2 Corinthians 5:7)

 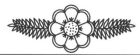

DAY 118	SU MO TU WE TH FR SA	How Do I Feel Today
	DATE: _____	

BREAKFAST	LUNCH	DINNER

SNACKS:

TOTAL CALORIES	GLASSES OF WATER	HOURS OF SLEEP

WEIGHT	BLOOD PRESSURE	BLOOD SUGAR

EXERCISE/ PHYSICAL ACTIVITY	SELF-CARE ACTIVITY

I will seek his will in all that I do, and he will show me which path to take.
(Proverbs 3:6)

DAY 119	SU MO TU WE TH FR SA DATE: _____	How Do I Feel Today

BREAKFAST	LUNCH	DINNER

SNACKS:

TOTAL CALORIES	GLASSES OF WATER	HOURS OF SLEEP

WEIGHT	BLOOD PRESSURE	BLOOD SUGAR

EXERCISE/ PHYSICAL ACTIVITY	SELF-CARE ACTIVITY

With God, all things are possible. (Luke 1:37)

 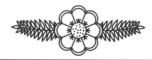

DAY 120

SU MO TU WE TH FR SA

DATE: _____

How Do I Feel Today

BREAKFAST	LUNCH	DINNER

SNACKS:

TOTAL CALORIES	GLASSES OF WATER	HOURS OF SLEEP

WEIGHT	BLOOD PRESSURE	BLOOD SUGAR

EXERCISE/ PHYSICAL ACTIVITY	SELF-CARE ACTIVITY

Whatever I ask in prayer, I will believe that I have received it, and it will be mine. (Mark 11:24)

 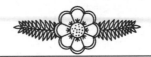

DAY 121

SU MO TU WE TH FR SA

DATE: _____

How Do I Feel Today

☐ ☐ ☐ ☐

BREAKFAST	LUNCH	DINNER

SNACKS:

TOTAL CALORIES	GLASSES OF WATER	HOURS OF SLEEP

WEIGHT	BLOOD PRESSURE	BLOOD SUGAR

EXERCISE/ PHYSICAL ACTIVITY	SELF-CARE ACTIVITY

Faith is the assurance of things hoped for, the conviction of things not seen. (Hebrews 11:1)

DAY 122

SU MO TU WE TH FR SA

DATE: _____

How Do I Feel Today

☐ ☐ ☐ ☐

BREAKFAST	LUNCH	DINNER

SNACKS:

TOTAL CALORIES	GLASSES OF WATER	HOURS OF SLEEP

WEIGHT	BLOOD PRESSURE	BLOOD SUGAR

EXERCISE/ PHYSICAL ACTIVITY	SELF-CARE ACTIVITY

Without faith it is impossible to please God, for whoever would draw near to God must believe that he exists and that he rewards those who seek him. (Hebrews 11:6)

 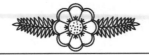

DAY 123

SU MO TU WE TH FR SA

DATE: _____

How Do I Feel Today

BREAKFAST	LUNCH	DINNER

SNACKS:

TOTAL CALORIES	GLASSES OF WATER	HOURS OF SLEEP

WEIGHT	BLOOD PRESSURE	BLOOD SUGAR

EXERCISE/ PHYSICAL ACTIVITY	SELF-CARE ACTIVITY

Faith comes from hearing, and hearing through the word of Christ.
(Romans 10:17)

 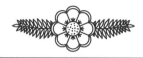

DAY 124	SU MO TU WE TH FR SA DATE: _____	How Do I Feel Today

BREAKFAST	LUNCH	DINNER

SNACKS:

TOTAL CALORIES	GLASSES OF WATER	HOURS OF SLEEP

WEIGHT	BLOOD PRESSURE	BLOOD SUGAR

EXERCISE/ PHYSICAL ACTIVITY	SELF-CARE ACTIVITY

Whatever I ask in prayer, I will receive it, because I have faith in Christ.
(Matthew 21:22)

 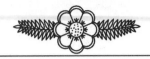

DAY 125

SU MO TU WE TH FR SA

DATE: _____

How Do I Feel Today

BREAKFAST	LUNCH	DINNER

SNACKS:

TOTAL CALORIES	GLASSES OF WATER	HOURS OF SLEEP

WEIGHT	BLOOD PRESSURE	BLOOD SUGAR

EXERCISE/ PHYSICAL ACTIVITY	SELF-CARE ACTIVITY

Love bears all things, believes all things, hopes all things, endures all things.
(1 Corinthians 13:7)

DAY 126	SU MO TU WE TH FR SA DATE: _____	How Do I Feel Today

BREAKFAST	LUNCH	DINNER

SNACKS:

TOTAL CALORIES	GLASSES OF WATER	HOURS OF SLEEP

WEIGHT	BLOOD PRESSURE	BLOOD SUGAR

EXERCISE/ PHYSICAL ACTIVITY	SELF-CARE ACTIVITY

I am a child of God.
(1 John 3:1)

 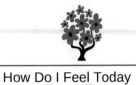

DAY 127	SU MO TU WE TH FR SA DATE: _____	How Do I Feel Today

BREAKFAST	LUNCH	DINNER

SNACKS:

TOTAL CALORIES	GLASSES OF WATER	HOURS OF SLEEP

WEIGHT	BLOOD PRESSURE	BLOOD SUGAR

EXERCISE/ PHYSICAL ACTIVITY	SELF-CARE ACTIVITY

God is love, and whoever abides in love abides in Christ, and Christ abides in him.
(1 John 4:16)

DAY 128	SU MO TU WE TH FR SA DATE: _____	How Do I Feel Today

BREAKFAST	LUNCH	DINNER

SNACKS:

TOTAL CALORIES	GLASSES OF WATER	HOURS OF SLEEP

WEIGHT	BLOOD PRESSURE	BLOOD SUGAR

EXERCISE/ PHYSICAL ACTIVITY	SELF-CARE ACTIVITY

The Lord gives strength to his people; the Lord blesses his people with peace. (Psalm 29:11)

 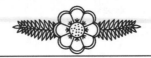

DAY 129

SU MO TU WE TH FR SA

DATE: _____

How Do I Feel Today

BREAKFAST	LUNCH	DINNER

SNACKS:

TOTAL CALORIES	GLASSES OF WATER	HOURS OF SLEEP

WEIGHT	BLOOD PRESSURE	BLOOD SUGAR

EXERCISE/ PHYSICAL ACTIVITY	SELF-CARE ACTIVITY

A friend loves at all times, and a brother is born for adversity.
(Proverbs 17:17)

DAY 130	SU MO TU WE TH FR SA DATE: _____	How Do I Feel Today

BREAKFAST	LUNCH	DINNER

SNACKS:

TOTAL CALORIES	GLASSES OF WATER	HOURS OF SLEEP

WEIGHT	BLOOD PRESSURE	BLOOD SUGAR

EXERCISE/ PHYSICAL ACTIVITY	SELF-CARE ACTIVITY

But God shows his love for me in that while I was still a sinner, Christ died for me.
(Romans 5:8)

 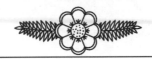

DAY 131

SU MO TU WE TH FR SA

DATE: _____

How Do I Feel Today

☐ ☐ ☐ ☐

BREAKFAST	LUNCH	DINNER

SNACKS:

TOTAL CALORIES	GLASSES OF WATER	HOURS OF SLEEP

WEIGHT	BLOOD PRESSURE	BLOOD SUGAR

EXERCISE/ PHYSICAL ACTIVITY	SELF-CARE ACTIVITY

So now, faith, hope, and love abide, these three; but the greatest of these is love.   (1 Corinthians 13:13)

DAY 132	SU MO TU WE TH FR SA DATE: _____	How Do I Feel Today

BREAKFAST	LUNCH	DINNER

SNACKS:

TOTAL CALORIES	GLASSES OF WATER	HOURS OF SLEEP

WEIGHT	BLOOD PRESSURE	BLOOD SUGAR

EXERCISE/ PHYSICAL ACTIVITY	SELF-CARE ACTIVITY

Love covers a multitude of sins.   (1 Peter 4:8)

 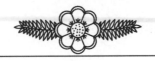

DAY 133

SU MO TU WE TH FR SA

DATE: _____

How Do I Feel Today

BREAKFAST	LUNCH	DINNER

SNACKS:

TOTAL CALORIES	GLASSES OF WATER	HOURS OF SLEEP

WEIGHT	BLOOD PRESSURE	BLOOD SUGAR

EXERCISE/ PHYSICAL ACTIVITY	SELF-CARE ACTIVITY

Above all, put on love, which binds everything together in perfect harmony. (Colossians 3:14)

 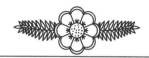

DAY 134	SU MO TU WE TH FR SA DATE: _____	How Do I Feel Today

BREAKFAST	LUNCH	DINNER

SNACKS:

TOTAL CALORIES	GLASSES OF WATER	HOURS OF SLEEP

WEIGHT	BLOOD PRESSURE	BLOOD SUGAR

EXERCISE/ PHYSICAL ACTIVITY	SELF-CARE ACTIVITY

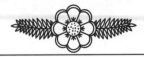

SU MO TU WE TH FR SA

DAY 135

DATE: _____

How Do I Feel Today

BREAKFAST	LUNCH	DINNER

SNACKS:

TOTAL CALORIES	GLASSES OF WATER	HOURS OF SLEEP

WEIGHT	BLOOD PRESSURE	BLOOD SUGAR

EXERCISE/ PHYSICAL ACTIVITY	SELF-CARE ACTIVITY

All that I do will be done in love.
(1 Corinthians 16:14)

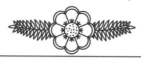

| DAY 136 | SU MO TU WE TH FR SA

DATE: _____ | How Do I Feel Today |

BREAKFAST	LUNCH	DINNER

SNACKS:

TOTAL CALORIES	GLASSES OF WATER	HOURS OF SLEEP

WEIGHT	BLOOD PRESSURE	BLOOD SUGAR

EXERCISE/ PHYSICAL ACTIVITY	SELF-CARE ACTIVITY

Love never ends. As for prophecies, they will pass away; as for tongues, they will cease; as for knowledge, it will pass away. (Hebrews 12: 2)

DAY 137

SU MO TU WE TH FR SA

DATE: _____

How Do I Feel Today

BREAKFAST	LUNCH	DINNER

SNACKS:

TOTAL CALORIES	GLASSES OF WATER	HOURS OF SLEEP

WEIGHT	BLOOD PRESSURE	BLOOD SUGAR

EXERCISE/ PHYSICAL ACTIVITY	SELF-CARE ACTIVITY

The Lord is faithful. He will establish me and guard me against the evil one. (2 Thessalonians 3:3)

 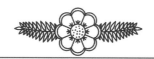

DAY 138	SU MO TU WE TH FR SA DATE: _____	How Do I Feel Today

BREAKFAST	LUNCH	DINNER

SNACKS:

TOTAL CALORIES	GLASSES OF WATER	HOURS OF SLEEP

WEIGHT	BLOOD PRESSURE	BLOOD SUGAR

EXERCISE/ PHYSICAL ACTIVITY	SELF-CARE ACTIVITY

The Lord is my strength and my song; he has become my salvation.
(Psalm 118:14)

 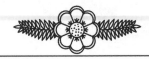

DAY 139

SU MO TU WE TH FR SA

DATE: _____

How Do I Feel Today

BREAKFAST	LUNCH	DINNER

SNACKS:

TOTAL CALORIES	GLASSES OF WATER	HOURS OF SLEEP

WEIGHT	BLOOD PRESSURE	BLOOD SUGAR

EXERCISE/ PHYSICAL ACTIVITY	SELF-CARE ACTIVITY

Even though I walk through the valley of the shadow of death, I will fear no evil,
for you are with me; your rod and your staff, they comfort me.   (Psalm 23:4)

DAY 140

SU MO TU WE TH FR SA

DATE: _____

How Do I Feel Today

☐ ☐ ☐ ☐

BREAKFAST	LUNCH	DINNER

SNACKS:

TOTAL CALORIES	GLASSES OF WATER	HOURS OF SLEEP

WEIGHT	BLOOD PRESSURE	BLOOD SUGAR

EXERCISE/ PHYSICAL ACTIVITY	SELF-CARE ACTIVITY

But you, Lord, are a shield around me, my glory, the One who lifts my head up high.
(Psalm 3:3)

DAY 141

SU MO TU WE TH FR SA

DATE: _____

How Do I Feel Today

BREAKFAST	LUNCH	DINNER

SNACKS:

TOTAL CALORIES	GLASSES OF WATER	HOURS OF SLEEP

WEIGHT	BLOOD PRESSURE	BLOOD SUGAR

EXERCISE/ PHYSICAL ACTIVITY	SELF-CARE ACTIVITY

May the Lord give strength to his people! May the Lord bless his people with peace!
(Psalm 29:11)

DAY 142	SU MO TU WE TH FR SA	How Do I Feel Today

DATE: _____

BREAKFAST	LUNCH	DINNER

SNACKS:

TOTAL CALORIES	GLASSES OF WATER	HOURS OF SLEEP

WEIGHT	BLOOD PRESSURE	BLOOD SUGAR

EXERCISE/ PHYSICAL ACTIVITY	SELF-CARE ACTIVITY

The Sovereign Lord gives me strength. He makes me sure-footed as a deer and keeps me safe on the mountains. (Habakkuk 3:19)

 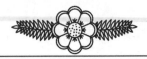

DAY 143

SU MO TU WE TH FR SA

DATE: _____

How Do I Feel Today

BREAKFAST	LUNCH	DINNER

SNACKS:

TOTAL CALORIES	GLASSES OF WATER	HOURS OF SLEEP

WEIGHT	BLOOD PRESSURE	BLOOD SUGAR

EXERCISE/ PHYSICAL ACTIVITY	SELF-CARE ACTIVITY

God is my refuge and strength, a very present help in trouble.
(Psalm 46:1)

DAY 144

SU MO TU WE TH FR SA

DATE: _____

How Do I Feel Today

BREAKFAST	LUNCH	DINNER

SNACKS:

TOTAL CALORIES	GLASSES OF WATER	HOURS OF SLEEP

WEIGHT	BLOOD PRESSURE	BLOOD SUGAR

EXERCISE/ PHYSICAL ACTIVITY	SELF-CARE ACTIVITY

This day is holy to the Lord. I will not be grieved, for the joy of the Lord is my strength.
(Nehemiah 8:10)

DAY 145

SU MO TU WE TH FR SA

DATE: _____

How Do I Feel Today

BREAKFAST	LUNCH	DINNER

SNACKS:

TOTAL CALORIES	GLASSES OF WATER	HOURS OF SLEEP

WEIGHT	BLOOD PRESSURE	BLOOD SUGAR

EXERCISE/ PHYSICAL ACTIVITY	SELF-CARE ACTIVITY

His grace is sufficient for me, for His power is made perfect in weakness.
(2 Corinthians 12:9)

 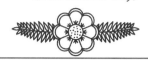

| DAY 146 | SU MO TU WE TH FR SA

DATE: _____ | How Do I Feel Today |

BREAKFAST	LUNCH	DINNER

SNACKS:

TOTAL CALORIES	GLASSES OF WATER	HOURS OF SLEEP

WEIGHT	BLOOD PRESSURE	BLOOD SUGAR

EXERCISE/ PHYSICAL ACTIVITY	SELF-CARE ACTIVITY

I will boast all the more gladly of my weaknesses, so that the power of Christ may rest upon me.
(2 Corinthians 12:9)

DAY 147

SU MO TU WE TH FR SA

DATE: _____

How Do I Feel Today

☐ ☐ ☐ ☐

BREAKFAST	LUNCH	DINNER

SNACKS:

TOTAL CALORIES	GLASSES OF WATER	HOURS OF SLEEP

WEIGHT	BLOOD PRESSURE	BLOOD SUGAR

EXERCISE/ PHYSICAL ACTIVITY	SELF-CARE ACTIVITY

My flesh and my heart may fail, but God is the strength of my heart and my portion forever.
(Psalm 73:26)

 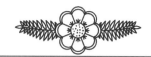

DAY 148

SU MO TU WE TH FR SA

DATE: _____

How Do I Feel Today

BREAKFAST	LUNCH	DINNER

SNACKS:

TOTAL CALORIES	GLASSES OF WATER	HOURS OF SLEEP

WEIGHT	BLOOD PRESSURE	BLOOD SUGAR

EXERCISE/ PHYSICAL ACTIVITY	SELF-CARE ACTIVITY

I will be strong and courageous, because my hope is in the Lord!
(Psalm 31:24)

DAY 149

SU MO TU WE TH FR SA

DATE: _____

How Do I Feel Today

BREAKFAST	LUNCH	DINNER

SNACKS:

TOTAL CALORIES	GLASSES OF WATER	HOURS OF SLEEP

WEIGHT	BLOOD PRESSURE	BLOOD SUGAR

EXERCISE/ PHYSICAL ACTIVITY	SELF-CARE ACTIVITY

The Lord is my light and my salvation; whom shall I fear? The Lord is the strength of my life; of whom shall I be afraid?   (Psalm 27:1)

 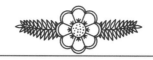

DAY 150	SU MO TU WE TH FR SA DATE: _____	How Do I Feel Today

BREAKFAST	LUNCH	DINNER

SNACKS:

TOTAL CALORIES	GLASSES OF WATER	HOURS OF SLEEP

WEIGHT	BLOOD PRESSURE	BLOOD SUGAR

EXERCISE/ PHYSICAL ACTIVITY	SELF-CARE ACTIVITY

He gives strength to the weary and increases the power of the weak.
(Isaiah 40:29)

DAY 151

SU MO TU WE TH FR SA

DATE: _____

How Do I Feel Today

BREAKFAST	LUNCH	DINNER

SNACKS:

TOTAL CALORIES	GLASSES OF WATER	HOURS OF SLEEP

WEIGHT	BLOOD PRESSURE	BLOOD SUGAR

EXERCISE/ PHYSICAL ACTIVITY	SELF-CARE ACTIVITY

I will trust, and will not be afraid; for the Lord God is my strength and my song, and he has become my salvation. (Isaiah 12:2)

DAY 152

SU MO TU WE TH FR SA

DATE: _____

How Do I Feel Today

☐ ☐ ☐ ☐

BREAKFAST	LUNCH	DINNER

SNACKS:

TOTAL CALORIES	GLASSES OF WATER	HOURS OF SLEEP

WEIGHT	BLOOD PRESSURE	BLOOD SUGAR

EXERCISE/ PHYSICAL ACTIVITY	SELF-CARE ACTIVITY

Surely your goodness and love will follow me all the days of my life,
and I will dwell in the house of the Lord for ever.   (Psalm 23:6)

 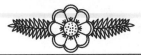

DAY 153

SU MO TU WE TH FR SA

DATE: _____

How Do I Feel Today

☐ ☐ ☐ ☐

BREAKFAST	LUNCH	DINNER

SNACKS:

TOTAL CALORIES	GLASSES OF WATER	HOURS OF SLEEP

WEIGHT	BLOOD PRESSURE	BLOOD SUGAR

EXERCISE/ PHYSICAL ACTIVITY	SELF-CARE ACTIVITY

For the Lord my God is he who goes with me to fight for me against the enemy,
to give me the victory. (Deuteronomy 20:4)

DAY 154

SU MO TU WE TH FR SA

DATE: _____

How Do I Feel Today

BREAKFAST	LUNCH	DINNER

SNACKS:

TOTAL CALORIES	GLASSES OF WATER	HOURS OF SLEEP

WEIGHT	BLOOD PRESSURE	BLOOD SUGAR

EXERCISE/ PHYSICAL ACTIVITY	SELF-CARE ACTIVITY

I am strong in the Lord and in His mighty power.
(Ephesians 6:10)

DAY 155

SU MO TU WE TH FR SA

DATE: _____

How Do I Feel Today

BREAKFAST	LUNCH	DINNER

SNACKS:

TOTAL CALORIES	GLASSES OF WATER	HOURS OF SLEEP

WEIGHT	BLOOD PRESSURE	BLOOD SUGAR

EXERCISE/ PHYSICAL ACTIVITY	SELF-CARE ACTIVITY

Those who wait for the Lord shall renew their strength; they shall mount up with wings like eagles;
They shall run and not be weary; they shall walk and not faint.   (Isaiah 40:31)

DAY 156	SU MO TU WE TH FR SA DATE: _____	How Do I Feel Today

BREAKFAST	LUNCH	DINNER

SNACKS:

TOTAL CALORIES	GLASSES OF WATER	HOURS OF SLEEP

WEIGHT	BLOOD PRESSURE	BLOOD SUGAR

EXERCISE/ PHYSICAL ACTIVITY	SELF-CARE ACTIVITY

I will be strong and courageous. I will not fear, for the Lord my God goes with me.
He will never leave me or forsake me. (Deuteronomy 31:6)

 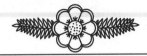

DAY 157	SU MO TU WE TH FR SA DATE: _____	How Do I Feel Today

BREAKFAST	LUNCH	DINNER

SNACKS:

TOTAL CALORIES	GLASSES OF WATER	HOURS OF SLEEP

WEIGHT	BLOOD PRESSURE	BLOOD SUGAR

EXERCISE/ PHYSICAL ACTIVITY	SELF-CARE ACTIVITY

I will not fear, for the Lord is with me; I will not be dismayed, for He is my God; He will strengthen me and help me, he will uphold me with His righteous right hand. (Isaiah 41:10)

DAY 158	SU MO TU WE TH FR SA DATE: _____	How Do I Feel Today

BREAKFAST	LUNCH	DINNER

SNACKS:

TOTAL CALORIES	GLASSES OF WATER	HOURS OF SLEEP

WEIGHT	BLOOD PRESSURE	BLOOD SUGAR

EXERCISE/ PHYSICAL ACTIVITY	SELF-CARE ACTIVITY

I can do all things through Christ who strengthens me.
(Philippians 4:13)

DAY 159

SU MO TU WE TH FR SA

DATE: _____

How Do I Feel Today

BREAKFAST	LUNCH	DINNER

SNACKS:

TOTAL CALORIES	GLASSES OF WATER	HOURS OF SLEEP

WEIGHT	BLOOD PRESSURE	BLOOD SUGAR

EXERCISE/ PHYSICAL ACTIVITY	SELF-CARE ACTIVITY

Since, I have been raised up with Christ, I will set my heart on things above,
where Christ is, seated at the right hand of God. (Colossians 3:1)

 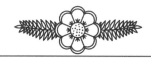

DAY 160

SU MO TU WE TH FR SA

DATE: _____

How Do I Feel Today

BREAKFAST	LUNCH	DINNER

SNACKS:

TOTAL CALORIES	GLASSES OF WATER	HOURS OF SLEEP

WEIGHT	BLOOD PRESSURE	BLOOD SUGAR

EXERCISE/ PHYSICAL ACTIVITY	SELF-CARE ACTIVITY

May the eyes of my understanding be enlightened; so that I may know what is the hope of His calling, and what are the riches of the glory of His inheritance in the saints. (Ephesians 1:18)

 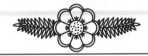

DAY 161	SU MO TU WE TH FR SA

DATE: _____

How Do I Feel Today

☐ ☐ ☐ ☐

BREAKFAST	LUNCH	DINNER

SNACKS:

TOTAL CALORIES	GLASSES OF WATER	HOURS OF SLEEP

WEIGHT	BLOOD PRESSURE	BLOOD SUGAR

EXERCISE/ PHYSICAL ACTIVITY	SELF-CARE ACTIVITY

I will not focus on the things which are seen, but on the things which are not seen. For the things which are seen are temporary, but the things which are not seen are eternal. (2 Corinthians 4:17-18)

 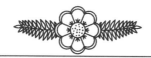

DAY 162

SU MO TU WE TH FR SA

DATE: _____

How Do I Feel Today

BREAKFAST	LUNCH	DINNER

SNACKS:

TOTAL CALORIES	GLASSES OF WATER	HOURS OF SLEEP

WEIGHT	BLOOD PRESSURE	BLOOD SUGAR

EXERCISE/ PHYSICAL ACTIVITY	SELF-CARE ACTIVITY

He who sows to the Spirit will of the Spirit reap everlasting life. (Galatians 6:8)

 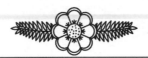

DAY 163

SU MO TU WE TH FR SA

DATE: _____

How Do I Feel Today

☐ ☐ ☐ ☐

BREAKFAST	LUNCH	DINNER

SNACKS:

TOTAL CALORIES	GLASSES OF WATER	HOURS OF SLEEP

WEIGHT	BLOOD PRESSURE	BLOOD SUGAR

EXERCISE/ PHYSICAL ACTIVITY	SELF-CARE ACTIVITY

I am a child of God; and it has not yet been revealed what I will be, but I know that when He is revealed, I will be like Him, for I will see Him as He is. (1 John 3:2)

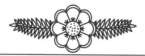

DAY 164	SU MO TU WE TH FR SA DATE: _____	How Do I Feel Today

BREAKFAST	LUNCH	DINNER

SNACKS:

TOTAL CALORIES	GLASSES OF WATER	HOURS OF SLEEP

WEIGHT	BLOOD PRESSURE	BLOOD SUGAR

EXERCISE/ PHYSICAL ACTIVITY	SELF-CARE ACTIVITY

My hope is in Christ.
(Psalm 39:7)

DAY 165

SU MO TU WE TH FR SA

DATE: _____

How Do I Feel Today

BREAKFAST	LUNCH	DINNER

SNACKS:

TOTAL CALORIES	GLASSES OF WATER	HOURS OF SLEEP

WEIGHT	BLOOD PRESSURE	BLOOD SUGAR

EXERCISE/ PHYSICAL ACTIVITY	SELF-CARE ACTIVITY

For God knew his people in advance, and he chose them to become like his Son, so that his Son would be the firstborn among many brothers and sisters. (Romans 8:29)

DAY 166

SU MO TU WE TH FR SA

DATE: _____

How Do I Feel Today

BREAKFAST	LUNCH	DINNER

SNACKS:

TOTAL CALORIES	GLASSES OF WATER	HOURS OF SLEEP

WEIGHT	BLOOD PRESSURE	BLOOD SUGAR

EXERCISE/ PHYSICAL ACTIVITY	SELF-CARE ACTIVITY

For his Spirit joins with our spirit to affirm that we are God's children, since we are His children, we are his heirs, and joint heirs with Christ Jesus.   (Romans 8:16-17)

 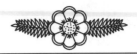

DAY 167

SU MO TU WE TH FR SA

DATE: _____

How Do I Feel Today

☐ ☐ ☐ ☐

BREAKFAST	LUNCH	DINNER

SNACKS:

TOTAL CALORIES	GLASSES OF WATER	HOURS OF SLEEP

WEIGHT	BLOOD PRESSURE	BLOOD SUGAR

EXERCISE/ PHYSICAL ACTIVITY	SELF-CARE ACTIVITY

Christ is living in me, giving me the hope of glory. (Colossians 1:27)

 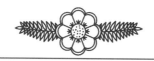

DAY 168	SU MO TU WE TH FR SA DATE: _____	How Do I Feel Today

BREAKFAST	LUNCH	DINNER

SNACKS:

TOTAL CALORIES	GLASSES OF WATER	HOURS OF SLEEP

WEIGHT	BLOOD PRESSURE	BLOOD SUGAR

EXERCISE/ PHYSICAL ACTIVITY	SELF-CARE ACTIVITY

He who has begun a good work in me will complete it until the day of Jesus Christ.
(Philippians 1:6)

DAY 169

SU MO TU WE TH FR SA

DATE: _____

How Do I Feel Today

BREAKFAST	LUNCH	DINNER

SNACKS:

TOTAL CALORIES	GLASSES OF WATER	HOURS OF SLEEP

WEIGHT	BLOOD PRESSURE	BLOOD SUGAR

EXERCISE/ PHYSICAL ACTIVITY	SELF-CARE ACTIVITY

I consider that the sufferings of this present time are not worthy to be compared with the glory, which shall be revealed in us. (Romans 8:18)

 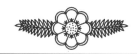

DAY 170	SU MO TU WE TH FR SA DATE: _____	How Do I Feel Today

BREAKFAST	LUNCH	DINNER

SNACKS:

TOTAL CALORIES	GLASSES OF WATER	HOURS OF SLEEP

WEIGHT	BLOOD PRESSURE	BLOOD SUGAR

EXERCISE/ PHYSICAL ACTIVITY	SELF-CARE ACTIVITY

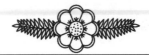

DAY 171

SU MO TU WE TH FR SA

DATE: _____

How Do I Feel Today

BREAKFAST	LUNCH	DINNER

SNACKS:

TOTAL CALORIES	GLASSES OF WATER	HOURS OF SLEEP

WEIGHT	BLOOD PRESSURE	BLOOD SUGAR

EXERCISE/ PHYSICAL ACTIVITY	SELF-CARE ACTIVITY

Fear not, for I have redeemed you; I have called you by your name; you are Mine, says the Lord.
(Isaiah 43:1)

DAY 172	SU MO TU WE TH FR SA DATE: _____	How Do I Feel Today

BREAKFAST	LUNCH	DINNER

SNACKS:

TOTAL CALORIES	GLASSES OF WATER	HOURS OF SLEEP

WEIGHT	BLOOD PRESSURE	BLOOD SUGAR

EXERCISE/ PHYSICAL ACTIVITY	SELF-CARE ACTIVITY

When I go through deep waters, He will be with me.
When I go through rivers of difficulty, I will not drown. (Isaiah 43:2)

DAY 173

SU MO TU WE TH FR SA

DATE: _____

How Do I Feel Today

BREAKFAST	LUNCH	DINNER

SNACKS:

TOTAL CALORIES	GLASSES OF WATER	HOURS OF SLEEP

WEIGHT	BLOOD PRESSURE	BLOOD SUGAR

EXERCISE/ PHYSICAL ACTIVITY	SELF-CARE ACTIVITY

When I walk through the fire of oppression, I will not be burned up;
the flames will not consume me. (Isaiah 43:2)

DAY 174	SU MO TU WE TH FR SA DATE: _____	How Do I Feel Today

BREAKFAST	LUNCH	DINNER

SNACKS:

TOTAL CALORIES	GLASSES OF WATER	HOURS OF SLEEP

WEIGHT	BLOOD PRESSURE	BLOOD SUGAR

EXERCISE/ PHYSICAL ACTIVITY	SELF-CARE ACTIVITY

The faithful love of the Lord never ends! His mercies never cease. They are new every morning.
Great is His faithfulness.   (Lamentations 3:22)

DAY 175

SU MO TU WE TH FR SA

DATE: _____

How Do I Feel Today

☐ ☐ ☐ ☐

BREAKFAST	LUNCH	DINNER

SNACKS:

TOTAL CALORIES	GLASSES OF WATER	HOURS OF SLEEP

WEIGHT	BLOOD PRESSURE	BLOOD SUGAR

EXERCISE/ PHYSICAL ACTIVITY	SELF-CARE ACTIVITY

Blessed is the one who trusts in the Lord, whose confidence is in him. (Jeremiah 17:7)

 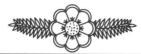

DAY 176	SU MO TU WE TH FR SA DATE: _____	How Do I Feel Today

BREAKFAST	LUNCH	DINNER

SNACKS:

TOTAL CALORIES	GLASSES OF WATER	HOURS OF SLEEP

WEIGHT	BLOOD PRESSURE	BLOOD SUGAR

EXERCISE/ PHYSICAL ACTIVITY	SELF-CARE ACTIVITY

If we hope for what we do not see, we eagerly wait for it with perseverance.
(Romans 8:25)

DAY 177

SU MO TU WE TH FR SA

DATE: _____

How Do I Feel Today

☐ ☐ ☐ ☐

BREAKFAST	LUNCH	DINNER

SNACKS:

TOTAL CALORIES	GLASSES OF WATER	HOURS OF SLEEP

WEIGHT	BLOOD PRESSURE	BLOOD SUGAR

EXERCISE/ PHYSICAL ACTIVITY	SELF-CARE ACTIVITY

Hope does not disappoint, because the love of God has been poured out in our hearts by the Holy Spirit who was given to us. (Romans 5:5)

 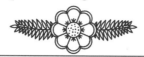

DAY 178

SU MO TU WE TH FR SA

DATE: _____

How Do I Feel Today

BREAKFAST	LUNCH	DINNER

SNACKS:

TOTAL CALORIES	GLASSES OF WATER	HOURS OF SLEEP

WEIGHT	BLOOD PRESSURE	BLOOD SUGAR

EXERCISE/ PHYSICAL ACTIVITY	SELF-CARE ACTIVITY

Jesus is able, once and forever, to save those who come to God through him.
He lives forever to intercede with God on their behalf. (Hebrews 7:25)

DAY 179

SU MO TU WE TH FR SA

DATE: _____

How Do I Feel Today

BREAKFAST	LUNCH	DINNER

SNACKS:

TOTAL CALORIES	GLASSES OF WATER	HOURS OF SLEEP

WEIGHT	BLOOD PRESSURE	BLOOD SUGAR

EXERCISE/ PHYSICAL ACTIVITY	SELF-CARE ACTIVITY

The Lord is my light and my salvation; whom shall I fear?
The Lord is the strength of my life; of whom shall I be afraid? (Psalm 27:1)

 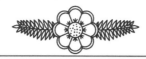

DAY 180	SU MO TU WE TH FR SA DATE: _____	How Do I Feel Today

BREAKFAST	LUNCH	DINNER

SNACKS:

TOTAL CALORIES	GLASSES OF WATER	HOURS OF SLEEP

WEIGHT	BLOOD PRESSURE	BLOOD SUGAR

EXERCISE/ PHYSICAL ACTIVITY	SELF-CARE ACTIVITY

The Lord my God is with me, the Mighty Warrior who saves. He takes great delight in me.
(Zephaniah 3:17)

DAY 181

SU MO TU WE TH FR SA

DATE: _____

How Do I Feel Today

BREAKFAST	LUNCH	DINNER

SNACKS:

TOTAL CALORIES	GLASSES OF WATER	HOURS OF SLEEP

WEIGHT	BLOOD PRESSURE	BLOOD SUGAR

EXERCISE/ PHYSICAL ACTIVITY	SELF-CARE ACTIVITY

Be strong and courageous. Do not fear or be in dread of them, for it is the Lord your God who goes with you. He will not leave you or forsake you. (Lamentations 3:22-23)

 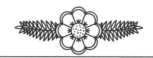

DAY 182	SU MO TU WE TH FR SA DATE: _____	How Do I Feel Today

BREAKFAST	LUNCH	DINNER

SNACKS:

TOTAL CALORIES	GLASSES OF WATER	HOURS OF SLEEP

WEIGHT	BLOOD PRESSURE	BLOOD SUGAR

EXERCISE/ PHYSICAL ACTIVITY	SELF-CARE ACTIVITY

Oh, taste and see that the Lord is good! Blessed is the man who takes refuge in him! (Psalm 34:8)

DAY 183

SU MO TU WE TH FR SA

DATE: _____

How Do I Feel Today

BREAKFAST	LUNCH	DINNER

SNACKS:

TOTAL CALORIES	GLASSES OF WATER	HOURS OF SLEEP

WEIGHT	BLOOD PRESSURE	BLOOD SUGAR

EXERCISE/ PHYSICAL ACTIVITY	SELF-CARE ACTIVITY

DAY 184

SU MO TU WE TH FR SA

DATE: _____

How Do I Feel Today

BREAKFAST	LUNCH	DINNER

SNACKS:

TOTAL CALORIES	GLASSES OF WATER	HOURS OF SLEEP

WEIGHT	BLOOD PRESSURE	BLOOD SUGAR

EXERCISE/ PHYSICAL ACTIVITY	SELF-CARE ACTIVITY

Fear not, for I am with you; be not dismayed, for I am your God; I will strengthen you, I will help you, I will uphold you with my righteous right hand.   (Isaiah 41:10)

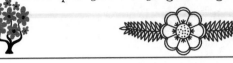

DAY 185

SU MO TU WE TH FR SA

DATE: _____

How Do I Feel Today

BREAKFAST	LUNCH	DINNER

SNACKS:

TOTAL CALORIES	GLASSES OF WATER	HOURS OF SLEEP

WEIGHT	BLOOD PRESSURE	BLOOD SUGAR

EXERCISE/ PHYSICAL ACTIVITY	SELF-CARE ACTIVITY

The Lord is my shepherd; I shall not want.
(Psalm 23:1)

 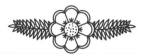

| DAY 186 | SU MO TU WE TH FR SA

DATE: _____ | How Do I Feel Today |
| --- | --- | --- |

BREAKFAST	LUNCH	DINNER

SNACKS:

TOTAL CALORIES	GLASSES OF WATER	HOURS OF SLEEP

WEIGHT	BLOOD PRESSURE	BLOOD SUGAR

EXERCISE/ PHYSICAL ACTIVITY	SELF-CARE ACTIVITY

God is within me, I will not fall; From the very break of day, God will protect me.
(Psalm 46:5)

DAY 187

SU MO TU WE TH FR SA

DATE: _____

How Do I Feel Today

BREAKFAST	LUNCH	DINNER

SNACKS:

TOTAL CALORIES	GLASSES OF WATER	HOURS OF SLEEP

WEIGHT	BLOOD PRESSURE	BLOOD SUGAR

EXERCISE/ PHYSICAL ACTIVITY	SELF-CARE ACTIVITY

Anyone who belongs to Christ has become a new person. The old life is gone; a new life has begun!
(2 Corinthians 5:17)

 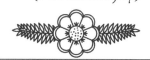

DAY 188	SU MO TU WE TH FR SA	How Do I Feel Today
	DATE: _____	😄 ☹️ 😔 😠 ☐ ☐ ☐ ☐

BREAKFAST	LUNCH	DINNER

SNACKS:

TOTAL CALORIES	GLASSES OF WATER	HOURS OF SLEEP

WEIGHT	BLOOD PRESSURE	BLOOD SUGAR

EXERCISE/ PHYSICAL ACTIVITY	SELF-CARE ACTIVITY

I sought the Lord, and he answered me; he delivered me from all my fears.
Those who look to him are radiant; their faces are never covered with shame. (Psalm 34:4-5)

DAY 189	SU MO TU WE TH FR SA DATE: _____	How Do I Feel Today

BREAKFAST	LUNCH	DINNER

SNACKS:

TOTAL CALORIES	GLASSES OF WATER	HOURS OF SLEEP

WEIGHT	BLOOD PRESSURE	BLOOD SUGAR

EXERCISE/ PHYSICAL ACTIVITY	SELF-CARE ACTIVITY

I took my troubles to the Lord; I cried out to him, and he answered my prayer.
(Psalm 120:1)

DAY 190	SU MO TU WE TH FR SA DATE: _____	How Do I Feel Today

BREAKFAST	LUNCH	DINNER

SNACKS:

TOTAL CALORIES	GLASSES OF WATER	HOURS OF SLEEP

WEIGHT	BLOOD PRESSURE	BLOOD SUGAR

EXERCISE/ PHYSICAL ACTIVITY	SELF-CARE ACTIVITY

I will lay aside every weight, and the sin which so easily beset me, and I will run with patience the race that is set before me. (Hebrews 12:1)

The End Point

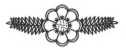

Current Stats

- Blood Pressure: _____
- Blood Sugar: _____
- Cholesterol: _____
- Weight: _____
- Thigh: _____
- Waist: _____
- Hips: _____
- BMI: _____

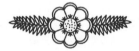

Overall Feelings Toward:

where you are at this point in your journey compared to where you were when you started and where you had expected to be at this point.

Reflections

I have fought a good fight, I have finished my course, I have kept the faith.
(2 Timothy 4:7)

Reflect on the goals that you have made at the beginning of your journey

Which goals did you accomplish?

Which goals did you not accomplish?

Explain Below...

Diet

Exercise

Weight Loss

Selfcare

Blood pressure, blood sugar, cholesterol levels etc.

Reflections on Goals

But none of these things move me, neither count I my life dear unto myself, so that I might finish my course with joy, to testify of the gospel of the grace of God.   (Acts 20:24)

Now that you have come to the end of this phase of your health, wellness and self-care journey, how has your perspective (concerning diet, exercise, weight loss, selfcare etc.) been affected by your experiences over the past 6 months?

Reflections

What are your goals for the next phase of your health,
wellness & selfcare journey?

Diet, exercise, weight loss, selfcare
Blood sugar, blood pressure & cholesterol levels etc.

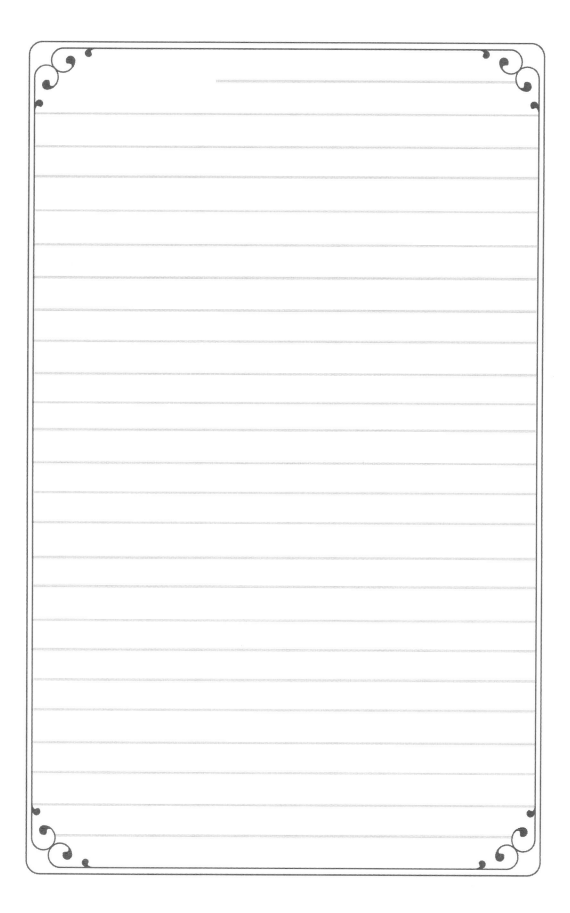

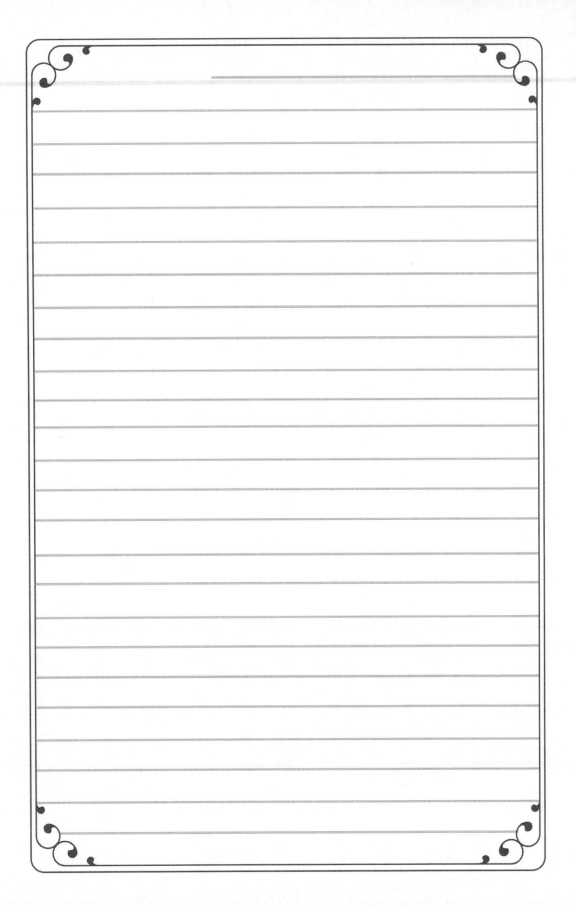

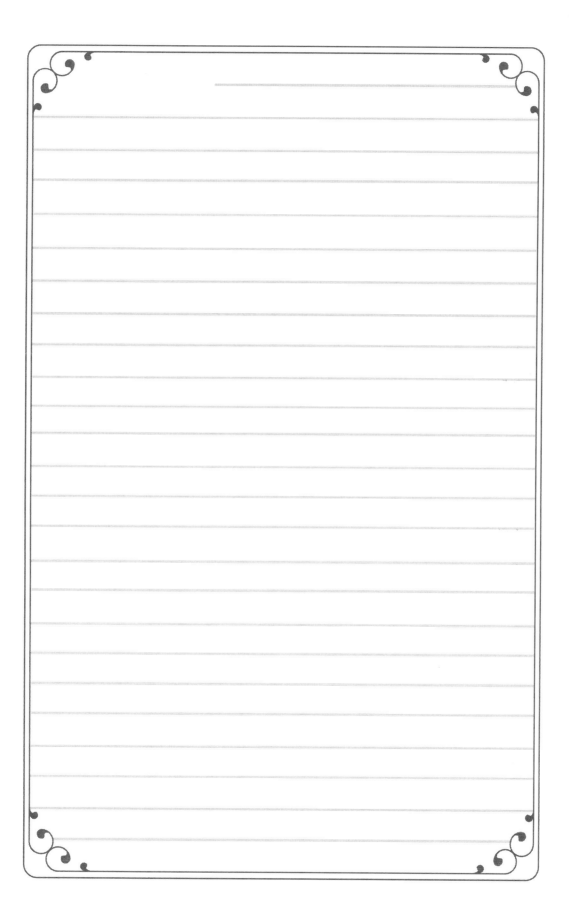

Made in United States
Orlando, FL
15 August 2022

21005221R00115